MASS MADE SIMPLE

MASS MADE SIMPLE

A Six-Week Journey into Bulking

Dan John

On Target Publications
Santa Cruz, California

Mass Made Simple
A Six-Week Journey into Bulking

Dan John

Copyright © 2011, Daniel Arthur John
ISBN: 978-1-931046-02-2

Photos taken at The Weight Room, Santa Cruz, California

Also by Dan John
Never Let Go: A Philosophy of Lifting, Living and Learning

15 14 13 12   2 3 4 5

On Target Publications
P. O. Box 1335
Aptos, CA 95001 USA
(888) 466-9185, Fax (831) 466-9183
info@otpbooks.com
www.otpbooks.com

Library of Congress Cataloging-in-Publication Data

John, Dan.
  Mass made simple : a six-week journey into bulking / Dan John.
     p. cm.
  ISBN 978-1-931046-02-2 (pbk.)
  1. Bodybuilding. 2. Muscle strength. 3. Weight training. I. Title.
  GV546.5.J64 2011
  796.41--dc22
                    2010054092

Contents

Disclaimer

The information contained herein is not intended to be a substitute for professional medical advice, diagnosis or treatment in any manner. Always seek the advice of your physician or other qualified health provider with any questions you may have regarding any medical condition or before engaging in any physical fitness plan.

My
"Overnight Success" in Mass Building
40 Pounds in Four Months

I didn't know it until I had been teaching for years, but a small decision in my youth had a massive impact on my life and athletic career. My birthday is about as late as you can get in August, and back then the cutoff date for starting school was September first.

As the youngest of six kids, and given the fact that nobody held their kids back when I was growing up, there was no question when I would march off to kindergarten. And nearly every day for the first month, I cried. I was the youngest in the class and far less mature.

Now, I must have loved tanks because everything I drew had tanks in it. One of my clearest memories of kindergarten, and frankly there are few, is my teacher asking me to draw something besides tanks. In fact, my mother had to meet with the teacher to convince me to do something besides draw tanks.

Even then, I guess, I was consumed with size and power. However, as a boy and, in this case anyway, as a Celt, maturation was a long way away. While the other boys with Mediterranean heritages hit a growth spurt in the sixth grade and had facial hair by the ninth, I was lucky enough to not hit puberty until well into high school. I played ninth grade football at 118 pounds and bulked up to 130 pounds as a sophomore. Honestly, I didn't shave daily until my mid-20s.

But I wanted to be an athlete. Fortunately, I had the right idea: I needed to lift weights. I caught the iron bug early when my brothers bought a weight set after our Aunt Florence died and left us a little money. We went to Sears and got the Ted Williams weight-lifting set with 110 pounds. Frankly, I doubted I would ever lift those big 15-pound plates. For the record, I did…and a lot more.

Every month, I would walk over to the corner pharmacy to see if *Strength and Health* had come in. It was the only information available, and it was perfect for me at that time. All the lifters were heroic, according to the articles, and lived on Hoffman's Hi-Proteen and drank the amazing Energol. Drugs were bad and clean living was the answer to all questions. Sure, I was young and believed it all—I only mastered cynicism in my 30s.

My lifting program was simple and I am amazed how much I still keep the same structure. The Southwood Program—see the extra stuff in the back of the book for the whole program, page 106—was perfect for me.

The program was based on this—

- Four lifts: *Power Clean, Front Squat, Military Press and Bench Press*
- A simple repetition scheme of 8–6-4
- We lifted in little groups. When we made all 18 repetitions with all four lifts, we moved up to the next weight during the next workout.

The descending-rep scheme was genius. It remains the cornerstone of my programming since 1971, and the four lifts are still the best movements I know for superior athletic performance.

Throughout high school, I had a love affair with the bench press. I saved up literally every quarter I had for over a year to buy an adjustable incline bench press. By this time, that original Ted Williams set had been expanded by "borrowing" plates from many of my neighbors; I could now get 132 ½ pounds on the bar. So, nearly every morning I went early to school to get some bench pressing in, then lifted after school with more bench pressing. At nights, I trained on our porch doing inclines and a host of other movements.

I got very strong in the bench press! How strong? Let's just say this: As a senior in high school I was stronger in the bench than when I was a senior in college, the high point man on the track and field team. I was so strong in the bench press, kids from other schools came to see me nail the big lifts.

And, I weighed 162 pounds as a senior. I could easily bench press double bodyweight, but I was only a lean, mean benching machine. When I finished high school, I knew I had to get bigger to compete with the heavier college discus. I knew, too, that I had to learn the Olympic lifts.

A guy at school told me there was an Olympic lifting meet in San Francisco, so I drove my Honda 200 up there to see what was going on. During a break in the competition, I went to use the restroom. It was down a small hallway and I had to make room for the guy coming out. His name was Dick Notmeyer, and he changed my life.

Dick owned the Pacifica Barbell Club just over the hill from me. I got to talk with him and he said I should join up, but the fee was high: 25 cents a week. From saving all those quarters to a now paying a quarter a week for a gym fee is too poetic to miss.

The following Monday, I pulled up to a house and started having doubts. In a minute or so, Dick opened the garage door and took me into his back room gym. It was small, but filled with equipment. Starting that day, I began doing the Olympic lifts. Three days a week, I was on the platform snatching and doing clean and jerks. Two days a week, I stepped to the rack to do front squats and jerks. That's right: two- to three-hour workouts just doing two lifts. Dick told me to "eat more" and "eat more protein." I did.

Four months later, I weighed 202 pounds—I went from 162 to 202 in four months. That's 10 pounds a month, two-and-a-half pounds a week, nearly half a pound a day. Go to a local fast-food place and order a quarter-pound burger. Imagine slapping 160 on those on your body in four months.

I came home one evening and my brother, Gary, was visiting. When I walked in, he looked up and said, "Holy shit." That's a bulking program.

Certainly, I grew larger in my career. Lifting as a 242-pound lifter, I often let my weight go up to as heavy as 273 before a contest. And, no, my friends, that is not a good plan. But, the gems of bulking have been laid out for you here—

- Mastery of the basic multi-joint barbell movements

- A commitment to getting stronger

- Real improvements come when you squat seriously (sorry!)

- Bulking is best done in a short period

- Finally, you need to be physically ready to bulk up. It's not something a nine-year-old can do!

And, one caveat: We will be talking about lean body mass here. Anyone, and it seems more like everyone, is bulking up today with a slothful lifestyle and massive amounts of cheap sugar. That's easy. Bulking up, especially for long-limbed guys, is tough.

Now, another caveat: I reported in the fall to Skyline College at 202. For the next nine months I held steady, although I rose to 204 pounds. How did I go from 162 to 202 in four months, then basically stop progress for nine months? Simple. I started track and field with Coach Bob Lualhauti and he had us doing some running, some bounding, some sprints, some throwing, some of this and some of that. In other words, if you decide to do more than just add lean body mass, your progress is going to stop.

There, a story and a warning. Now, follow me.

As to methods, there may be a million and then some, but principles are few. The man who grasps principles can successfully select his own methods. The man who tries methods, ignoring principles, is sure to have trouble. ~ **Emerson**

If you want methods for bulking, the fitness world is brimming with them. The conversation on forums usually goes like this (for ease of reading, I will actually capitalize words and attempt to spell them right, unlike the internets)—

Q: Hey, my good lads, I need a superior bulking program that will put on lots of weight quickly.

Answer from *lovetobulkupandcruise2*:

Try this: Work your legs on Monday, arms on Tuesday, chest and back on Wednesday, arms on Thursday, Friday just rest, arms on Saturday. Rest on Sunday, my brother in iron, as you will need it.

Answer from *biggestgunzinthelargermetropolitanareaofrawlinswyoming*:

Wow, that looks good, but I would switch Tuesday and Thursday.

Alas, it is only a slight exaggeration.

Breaking up the body into smaller parts, called splitting, is a method. Oh, it works and it can work very well. But that is just a "thing." Principle-based bulking is designed around four simple insights—

1. Everybody is the same, but just enough different to warrant some exploration.
2. Doing everything at once makes it difficult to discern what is working.
3. There is a need to spend time under a load.
4. There are some nutritional tweaks that work.

Everybody is the same, but just enough different to warrant some exploration.

In full candor, I believe in the absolute dignity of every human person. Having said that, I have also coached and played in sport for over four decades. Certainly, human size fits into a certain bell curve. As Nassim Taleb said, which I will paraphrase, if I told you that two people walking down the street had a sum of their heights at 12 feet, most people would get the idea that each of them was probably around six feet, give or take. It would be rare person who would guess a ten-footer and a two-footer were strolling together.

So, yes, we are all God's creatures endowed with certain inalienable rights and our mothers love us. Now, let's be honest: There are some people who are simply going to be stronger, faster and prettier than you and me and that is just the way it is. So, in discussing a bulking program, we have to accept some variations.

That's the problem with most methods of bulking. It is a template we simply step into and on Day One do this and that and this.

By the way, this method works! Except for some…so let's get back to the principle.

Stu McGill, the great Canadian back specialist, spent some quality time with me recently and noted I had a "Scottish Hip." Instantly, certain things made sense. Years ago, I was tested with a little machine that measured maximal poundage in certain lifting positions. At the quarter-squat position, I maxed out the machine at 1,400 (I'm not sure I could support it, but the system said I was pushing that amount). In the half-squat, I was at 255. The next guy was literally 405 in both positions.

I mentioned this story to Stu and he said, "Of course. That is why you do the Caber Toss and throw things. You are built for it." McGill is the expert here, and he told me to look at the popular sports of a region and how they tend to reflect the small but crucial differences in body structure.

To sum up: You have this structure. It's not going to change, and it is going to impact your bulking program. Long-limbed guys with narrow shoulders probably will struggle with double bodyweight squats for max reps.

And, there is more. I know guys who can treadmill for long periods of time. I get bored after touching all the buttons. I'm not going to be doing a lot of boring, repetitive stuff in my career because it is literally not in my nature. I work with athletes who can groove in on one thing and just keep doing it over and over.

Well, what about you? Can you sit at a terminal and work on the Williewank Proposal or whatever for 10 hours? Or do you have to be stimulated? The way you are wired to work has a huge impact on your training. With luck, a *One Size Fits All Program* might be perfect for you, but most people seem to have little luck beyond a few weeks with any program.

There is no question that the axiom *success leaves tracks* is true. Part of the issue with bulking is making sure those tracks take you on the right path.

Doing everything at once makes it difficult to discern what is working.

If there is one bit of clarity from my coaching career, it is this: **Keep It Simple, Stupid.** The KISS method is certainly just a cliché too many, but time and again it is the secret to success for most people.

Recently, I AGAIN had this conversation with an elite athlete who was injured. "How did you get hurt?" "Oh, well, we had this idea to do…" The athletic careers of so many amazing athletes have been brought to a halt by adding one new great idea that looked so promising on paper or on the 'net, trashing a bodypart in the process.

Here is a hint: *Stick with what was working and be very mindful of adding anything new.*

In bulking programs, very often the person is given a long list of things do, including food plans, supplements, secret voodoo stuff and lots of little other things. Well, which one works? Which one is counterproductive? I have tried many very expensive programs in the past, including one that set me back hundreds in supplements to train on an empty stomach then work to excess, but when one is mixing five or six or ten items, which one works?

Certain things make some people sick to their stomachs. Mix that with high-rep squats and you have the perfect recipe for a mess on the floor. You must take some time adding ingredients to the bulking recipe.

There is a need to spend time under a load.

To be honest, I think this is the most complex principle. Notice what I didn't say: You must do this exercise for this many reps and this many sets. Well, I will, but honestly the load can be any tool you want.

Barbells

Machines

Kettlebells

Sandbags

Rocks

Sleds

They all work. Now, some are obviously better for some things than the others, but the loading is the key. I made my biggest gains in bodyweight with weights that were not very heavy in hindsight, but they were killing me at the time. Why? Well, I had never done, for example, a front squat. The wrist flexibility issue alone was making my nights long. Add in all the other joints, the upright posture and the fact I had never done real squatting before added up to dead legs and tired arms and an aching back for a long time. My body responded, even to these relatively light loads, by exploding in growth.

Time is also a bit hazy, too. You can get freakishly big, if that's the way you are made, by doing just singles. I have never seen a waifish 800-pound deadlifter. The time it takes to deadlift a max attempt is far shorter than running a marathon, although you might feel the same after either finish. It does seem, by the eyeball test, that most guys who are long-limbed and a little taller need more reps and more time with a load in hand to gain size. If you are one of those 5' 2" fireplug-shaped guys, adding width might be pretty easy by just moving singles. If you are a 7' 2" NBA center, you need to spend some time with more repetitions.

There are great, simple ways of extending time under a load. Sadly, the two best are complexes and high-rep squats. Why sadly? They both make you feel awful! Now, if it is true that stomach upset is a sign of growth hormone release, at least you can feel happy that you are releasing GH for free.

There are some nutritional tweaks that work.

I feel bad for a lot of guys on bulking programs. In fact, in hindsight, I feel bad for me. I was on a gallon of milk a day to bulk up in the late 1970s. Later I found out I was lactose intolerant. That might have explained the explosiveness of my day (let's just say "I was gassy" and move on), and the huge acne cysts on my face. I was literally drinking a gallon of what was for me a kind of poison. Modern protein powders are miles ahead of what we had "back in the day," so this is much easier to deal with today.

I give this advice, over and over, for most people's goals—

Eat more protein.

Eat more fiber.

Take more fish oil.

And, that is exactly the advice I will give for each and every program I ever design for any sport or goal. But, we will go a bit farther. Instead of choking down as much as you can every day, we will build up to several very inventive techniques where we use the clock as much as we use the mouth to increase protein intake.

Creatine, for example, works wonders for some people and provides misery for others. In the traditional shot-gun approach to bulking, creatine would get added on Day One. We will do things different. I would rather give you a few days to test your personal response to creatine. Should you have no issues, stay the course. If cramping or distress appears, we know the culprit.

Isn't getting bigger/more massive/bulkier bad for your health?

For years I've promoted my *Do This!* list of 10 suggestions—originally I called it my Ten Commandments, but it seems this had been used before—as a simple toolkit for living, statistically, a long life. Here you go—

1. Don't smoke.
2. Wear your seatbelt. Use a helmet when appropriate, too.
3. Learn to fall… and recover!
4. Eat more protein.
5. Eat more fiber.
6. Drink more water.
7. Take fish oil capsules.
8. Floss your teeth.
9. Keep your joints healthy.
10. Build some muscle.

I have given this list to large groups, small groups, one-on-one, to nuns, to elite warriors, to NFL players, to Olympic-level athletes, to grandparents and kids. I think I can stand by each and every point, and I don't see any changes. Certainly, like the helmet issue, feel free to add or subtract.

One of my favorite stories reminds us about this point.

A young scholar is coming home from school and he has his satchel of books and a lofty air of intellect and superiority. He takes a small boat to get across the river that blocks his road home and the boatman asks a simple question, "What do you study in school?"

The young scholar won't deign to look the boatman in the eye. "Philosophy. Theology."

"Ah. Did they teach you to swim?"

"Of course not. We were discussing important questions."

"Too bad. The boat is sinking."

This little story reminds me of some of the other things, but overall, for the bulk of us, this list is pretty good. I see no reason how building lean body mass can be bad for you—in fact Number 10 underscores its value here. Now, having said that, just putting on *pounds* might be an issue.

Folks, and you know this, getting fat is easy. You have plenty of role models for how to do it. It seems consuming massive amounts of sugar-laded deep-fried carbs washed down with more sugary drinks while maintaining very low levels of movement seems to be the ticket here. I'm advising you NOT to do that, thank you very much. Truly adding lean body mass is difficult—not impossible, of course, but piling on lean body mass is hard to do.

In the next few years, and honestly we have been seeing the evidence pile up, the notion of healthy as in "healthy diet" and "healthy body" is going to see some revisionary thinking. A bulking program that builds lean body mass—I was recently told the measurement of lean body mass is practically all you need to determine the physical age, not the actual age of a person—might actually be as healthy as what we used to think about sprouts, wheat grass drinks and colonics.

One of the things the person seeking more mass will have to deal with is Fat Phobia.

It comes in two styles: first, and get ready for this, when one begins a mass program, somebody somewhere is going to say, "Well, it won't be any good if it is all fat." True. We have excellent fat-building protocols. Eat lots of sugars, sit around and watch television and drink lots of calories. True lean body mass-building is going to be a lot harder than that!

We also have a fear of fat in our foods. There has been a slow turning of the wheel concerning fats in foods in the past few years, but you really have to think about the image of the *Titanic* and the iceberg here. It's not turning very fast! I don't have a dog in this fight, but the hopeful mass gainer must be ready to hear the warnings about fat. There are a fair number of books published in the past few years with the words "Good," "Fat" and "Lies" in the title, and any of them are worth a look.

When it comes to gaining lean body mass, I have some thoughts, some insights, some programs and some clues to point you in the right direction. But, one thing has been proven to me over and over again with people striving to gain lean body mass: Some things will work for you and some things will not work for you.

As simple as that sounds, that is the overriding principle of this book. I have often noted that we are a lot like house plants in a funny way: If you have aphids in your house plants and you toss in 10 things to combat them and the aphids die (and maybe your house plant), well, what worked? What was poison? What helped? What hurt?

The mistake with most programs is what we used to call the Kitchen Sink approach, from the cliché *everything plus the kitchen sink*, and, no, I have no idea what it means either. On day one, you take this and that and this and that and do all of this stuff and that stuff, too. Within a week, you are a limping, barfing mess but your arms feel bigger. Well, what worked?

I know it sounds so simple but you have to add things a little at a time. Here is the upside, and I am giving you the secret of my four decades of sports performance: Once you know what works for you, it is always going to work for you to some degree. And, on the contrary, if something doesn't…my friend, run screaming from it.

Oh, it sounds so simple. But, like all truths, I said it was simple, not easy. Enjoy.

Let's Get Started: The Mental Side of Bulking

The Toolkit for Goal-Setting: The Key to Bulking

Eat your way to SUCCESS!!!

I think I could make a fortune with a book entitled *Eat Your Way to Success.* I love to browse bookstores through the diet, fitness and cooking sections and just feast on all the delicious options for food or not eating food. Everything makes you fat if you look through enough diet books. That same "thing" is also the cure for your fatness in a book one shelf away. Walk over to the personal success aisle and you can learn to talk to yourself until you have a million dollars. Rather than talk to yourself like the nice lady on the midnight bus from downtown, I suggest eating your way to success.

Honestly, the three best mental images I have for success involve eating. From what I have seen across the vast landscape of America, eating is not a rarity for many here in these United States. I have been elbowed by many a moo-mooed woman in a buffet line in Las Vegas and I have the war wounds to prove it. Sadly, my Frog, Elephant and Alpo Dog Food Diet might lose customers simply by the title. Every time I fly, I see an advertisement for something called The Cookie Diet. Now that can sell. Somehow, even if it was The All You Can Eat Frog, Elephant and Alpo Dog Food Diet, it still might not break the top 10 best-seller list.

If there is an axiom for a successful life and having any chance at achieving any goals, it would be the following—

"You can't do everything, but you can do something."

Let that sit before you for a moment. If I could do anything for my legacy to this fine planet earth, I would hope and pray it would be *Do Something.* For years at workshops I have been preaching my "secret" two words to success: *Show up.* I need to add "Do something," too.

In this approach to bulking, we are NOT going to do everything. We are going to add some basic things and see how the journey is taking you. But, you MUST do something: **SHOW UP!**

My favorite story about the magic of simply showing up happened in 1984. I was standing in line, after a long train ride to get to there and probably no real sleep in two days, to register for my intensive Turkish language class. Quick, imagine me standing in line because that is all I was doing. If you have ever stood in line, use that image if that is easier for you.

A guy behind the registration desk slammed a phone down, looked up at me and asked, "Do you want $1,500?" My answer…"Uh, yes." It turns out that another student who had been given a nice stipend just to show up decided to quit. I was given a check in the next three minutes for $1,500 for just standing in line.

If you want to be a national champion, you really need to get to the stadium on time. If you decide to get married, the ceremony starts at 11. Be there. Showing up is underrated as a life skills success clue.

Of course, showing up is only step one. Step two is to do something. When I counsel/mentor/coach/teach/help others in goal-setting, it often only takes a few minutes to outline a list of goals in every single area of life. Warning: Be careful about setting goals, because you may attain them. Almost every time I have had one of these goal-setting experiences, the person looks up and smiles from this sheet of paper, then the eyes go wide and the question comes forth, "Well, uh, what do I do?"

Do something.

Easy to type. Easy to read. And, actually, easy to do. The problem for most people is the magnitude of a goal seems to explode like the Big Bang before them. You want to get your college degree? Well, you have to register, get a parking pass, find the cafeteria, buy a school sweatshirt, find a lifetime friend to have several funny experiences with, go on a road trip, write and lose the Great American Novel, read a book simply from Cliff Notes…hey, you have a lot to do! For me, when someone says college, I have a refreshing mental image of fun, study and free time. Why the disconnect? Well, I've done it! Talk to people have done the goal you are interested in achieving, and, well, do what they say!

By following the path of generations of successful bulkers of the past, you are well on your way to success.

That is why I go to experts when I have a question. Years ago, as I often joke, I woke up fat. Many of you may understand that completely. Working two jobs, raising kids, mowing lawns, struggling with life and all the rest might just keep you from making excellent food and exercise decisions each and every day. And, one day, you wake up fat. So, I consulted a group of women called the 100-Pound Club. Each of the women had lost one hundred pounds through a variety of diets, exercise choices and attempts, and they discussed their findings freely. You see, they had been there. My friend Dave dropped one hundred pounds by simply making a new habit each month, from something as simple as drinking more water each day to walking each day. When it came time for serious goals, like running a half-marathon, his background of successfully nailing progressively harder goals led him across the finish line. If you want to learn about fat loss, ask a competitive bodybuilder. If you want to learn about persuasive speaking, read Lincoln or Churchill. If you want to learn the next step after showing up, listen to me. Let's do something!

To help you do something, we'll discuss my Frog, Elephant and Alpo Dog Food Diet.

The First Thing is To Do SOMETHING!

The first thing about getting things done is that there is always something, something big, sitting there that you don't want to do. Years ago, my wife Tiffini clued me in on how to deal with this.

"If you have to eat a plate of frogs, eat the biggest one first."

Hmmm? Listen, this "system" works. If you have to do something today involving a crappy phone call, an awful meeting or a visit to the IRS, schedule it first. I made a career as a strength coach by teaching people to FIRST do the stuff they don't want to do in the weightroom or in the field of play. Eat the biggest frog first.

Imagine a plate of frogs sitting before you. Now, imagine you will get a billion dollars for eating the whole plate. Would you do it? Or is your revulsion from eating our little frog friends so great you will pass on the billion? For me, I am going to shove those guys down my throat as fast as I can for a billion bucks. Yep, I have standards about food and drink, but I will take the billion, thank you very much.

Which one should you start with? Tiff tells us to reach in and grab the biggest one and swallow it down and, from there, none of the little ones will wiggle down as much.

So, rule one of "Do something" is to pick the worst thing you perceive of the new direction or decision and get rid of it. Surprisingly, it is usually not that bad. Moreover, the **relief**—breathe out, wipe your brow, relax your shoulders, smile again—of dealing with this first big frog makes the rest of the goal pretty easy. I have been there many times in my life. As a teacher, it is dealing with the crazy helicopter parent (the parent whirling constantly around the child); as a professional, it might be that task that just feels like labor pains and you can fill in the blank for yourself here. Find the big frog. Eat it.

So,
1. **Show up**
2. **Do something—Eat the Biggest Frog/Deal with the Toughest Issue First**

That is why we are going to emphasize the high-rep back squat in our bulking program from the first day to the last day. You are free to hate them, loathe them and perhaps never do them again the rest of your life, but, folks, in a bulking program, the high-rep back squat is the biggest frog I can find.

Wipe your palate clean from the frog juice, try a refreshing gelato, and let's get ready for the next meal: Elephant.

One of the oldest motivational clichés I know is this: *If you have to eat an elephant, start with one mouthful at a time.* In goal-setting success, you need to take small bites, but keep on biting! I can remember fondly when my daughter Kelly first began to learn to speak. I was overwhelmed, to be honest. Think about it: the days of the week, the names of the months, holidays, clocks, street signs, the presidents, the political system…there was so much to teach her!

She did fine. We didn't have one day to do it all. From preschool to elementary to high school to college, we ate a bit of the elephant every day. Trust me, if you can learn the days and the months, you can achieve your easier goals like adding some lean body mass.

So, *Do Something* comes in two flavors: frog (take on the ugliest task first) and elephant (attack a bit of the task every time you can). If your goal is to bulk up, have a few photos taken of you in your swimsuit. You will hate it. Learn to squat, if you don't already know how. A quality bulking program is going to be rough. But, what's your motivation? Successful people will almost always mention that it was a series of small goals, small changes that led to success. Now, let's talk about dog food.

The single best piece of diet advice I ever heard came from peak performance consultant Anthony Robbins. Robbins got his advice from one of his clients. It's called the Alpo Diet, and it goes like this: Invite a dozen friends over to your house. Tell them that by the end of the month you're going to lose 10 pounds. Tell them if you don't, you'll eat the can of Alpo in front of them.

For the next week, every time you feel the urge to take a piece of chocolate from the cubicle next to you, reread the contents of the Alpo can. If someone offers you something smothered in goo, open the Alpo can and take a good deep sniff.

The Robbins approach is based on the principle that most people would rather avoid pain than embrace joy or pleasure. I can sit you down and give you line after line, reason after reason about why making a life change or choice is going to really help you. I can show you movies of the new joy you will find once you fulfill your goals. And most people will ignore them. When you need some encouragement, crack open the can and sniff some Alpo and, for whatever reason, you'll tend to stick to the plan!

And, before you can say it, why don't people meet their goals? I have spent many hours at cafes, bars, bistros, cafeterias, libraries and corners of gyms walking people through pyramids, charts and schemes to achieve all manner of goals and, more often than not, they fail. Perhaps the answer is it's me. I seem to be the common denominator here.

And, I'm sure many people will take that option. Let's just blame Dan. I have broad shoulders, feel free to stand on them.

You see, motivation is a strange thing. Every person reading is familiar with some aspect of the Frog, Elephant and Alpo Dog Food Diet. None of this is news. Oh, this is going to be the cornerstone of your goal-achieving since this diet, simple as it may seem, is the foundation for every single goal ever achieved. Two parts of our success program, then, are this:

1. **Show up.**
2. **The Frog, Elephant and Alpo Dog Food Diet—Start with a tough task, keep chewing away and have something awful in mind if you fail.**

I don't want to walk away from the Alpo Diet too quickly. For years, I have argued that the best client a personal trainer can have would be someone like this—

- Recently divorced woman whose husband ran away with ex-best-friend, who is chubby
- High school reunion coming up where woman, ex-husband and ex-best-friend will all attend
- Old high school friend, who is also a billionaire now, really wants to "see her," as he had a crush on her all four years of school. His private jet will drop him off near his private helicopter at the reunion.

Now, with this woman I can make demands. "Twenty eggs a day." Fine. "Two workouts a day." I will do another on my own. "A pound of salmon for breakfast." Raw?

You see, pain brings clarity toward a goal. I would love to use pleasure as the crowbar to engage people to stick to their goals. I wish. There rarely seems enough pleasure out there to overcome the magic of cookies and creamy ice cream. The problem with goals and goal-setting is that it is hard to get someone to buy in to the promise of future pleasure to overcome momentary pain.

Next let's look at the mental toolkit and how it relates to this bulking plan.

First, you either bought, stole or borrowed this book. Congrats to you, you showed up.

You are already ahead of most of the people who want to simply wave a magic wand and get 20 pounds of lean body mass added on to their bodies.

Your task is simple. I'm going to ask that you show up at the weightroom a couple of times a week and train hard. I also want to add a few small additions to your diet. Some aspects will be hard and others will just be humoring me, even though you'll find some of these odd suggestions actually work.

The Frog? Well, that's going to be the back squat program. Sorry.

The Elephant? You need to follow the advice, do the workouts, ease up your other activities and move ahead one day at a time.

The Dog Food? That's up to you, my friend. When I decided to do the Velocity Diet, I started an extremely popular forum topic at *T-nation.com* and literally answered dozens of posts some days. I put it out there. If I failed that diet, it would have been a big deal and a real hit to my integrity. Part of the reason I was so successful with Dick Notmeyer's advice was that I was quickly running out of time to compete as a college athlete. I had to get bigger as fast as I could, and I poured all my energy into it. My dog food would have been the *woulda, coulda, shoulda* so many former high school athletes bore their friends and family with the rest of their lives. Please shuffle to *Glory Days* by Bruce Springsteen.

Pour your energy into these next few weeks of work. This is a familiar path; many have walked this before with great success. Now, it's your turn. Eat up!

Before we get too specific: Eat like an adult!

As much as I like talking about health, fitness, training and sports, I really don't like talking about food and diet very much. First, no matter what I say or what the research supports in the area of food and dietary practices, there is a mountain of evidence both scientific and experiential that will tout the opposite principle. Second, I was about to rant about something right from the beginning, but I have to hold it in.

Okay, I won't, so this is the point—

Honestly, seriously, you don't know what to do about food? Here is an idea: *Eat like an adult.* Stop eating fast food, stop eating kid's cereal, knock it off with all the sweets and comfort foods whenever your favorite show is not on when you want it on, ease up on the snacking and—don't act like you don't know this—eat vegetables and fruits more. Really, how difficult is this? Stop with the whining. Stop with the excuses. Act like an adult and stop eating like a television commercial. Grow up.

And, I would have stuck to this, save for one wonderful insight a few years ago. I was sitting in my basement watching a college football game. I am pretty sure the Florida Gators were playing someone, but I was focused on my meal. It was a t-bone steak, several eggs, some rye toast and a Scotch. Yes, you read that right.

You see, it was Saturday of my first week of the Velocity Diet. This meal was the first solid food I had eaten in six days. I lived on six protein shakes a day and a small sprinkling of supplements. The only thing missing from the V-Diet is food. The thing is, one begins to miss food after a while. As I finished up my meal, Tiffini looked at me, obviously concerned, and asked, "What's the matter?" "Huh?" Then I noticed tears were streaming down my cheeks. I couldn't get over it, and I would have laughed at anyone else with this response. Response?

Yes, I was having an emotional response to food. After all those years of making jokes about "comfort foods" and "eat like an adult," I was caught up in a swooning moment of literally instant depression at the notion that I wouldn't drink booze or eat anything fun again for seven days. I wasn't sobbing, but I was clearly emotionally ratcheted down.

Since that moment—and things got much better after that on the V-Diet by the way—I have a real appreciation for people who mention an odd relationship with food. I can understand how someone might sit and eat a box of cookies after an emotionally charged day (I would prefer you did not). I also understand why the comfort foods of youth might be attractive to someone without a great social network. I even have empathy for someone who might eat fast foods now because as a youth the family couldn't go out very much due to financial issues.

Good. Let's hug it out. Now, let's get back to the point: **Eat like an adult!**

Elaine St. James has made an industry out of living simply. My favorite of her books is *Simplify Your Life*. Her first point on "Your Health" is to simplify your eating habits. She and her husband decided to simplify life and discovered that making an honest effort at cutting meals shorter also led to a healthier diet.

She settled on two principles: one, no surprise here, eliminate the junk food. She goes on to discuss other basic options such as always splitting a restaurant meal when she goes go out. Two, they also ate fewer calories, less fat and cholesterol. They chose to drink water rather than all the rest of the options laden with cheap calories. Her diet plan is worthy of consideration for most people in most situations.

Breakfast
> Fruit in season, homemade granola, homemade oat muffins

Lunch
> Fresh fruit and/or vegetable crudités, with whole grain bread sandwiches made with sliced turkey or avocado, tomato and sprouts

Dinner
> Huge fresh salad or a cold soup, such as gazpacho, or hearty veggie soups and salad in winter, or steamed veggies and rice

On the path to simplicity and cutting back the time devoted to making meals, St. James has discovered a meal plan that most of us would recognize as healthy.

Others have addressed the simple meal structure in other ways. Tim Ferris, fellow RKC and author of the life-changing book, *The Four-Hour Work Week,* has four simple rules to follow:

1. *Avoid white carbohydrates.* That list would include breads, rice, pastas and the bulk of junk food. He also shuns potatoes and deep-fried breaded food.
2. *Eat the same foods over and over again.* He suggests splitting each meal into three parts—protein, legumes and vegetables—and filling the plate by covering one-third with each of the choices. The options include—

> **Proteins**
>
> **Egg whites with one whole egg for flavor**
>
> **Chicken breast or thigh**
>
> **Grass-fed organic beef**
>
> **Pork**
>
> **Legumes**
>
> **Lentils**
>
> **Black beans**
>
> **Pinto beans**
>
> **Vegetables**
>
> **Spinach**
>
> **Asparagus**
>
> **Peas**
>
> **Mixed vegetables**

3. *Don't drink calories.* St. James and nearly every other author agrees—

> **Drink water.**

4. *Have one cheat day.* Give yourself a break one day a week. Although some diet plans argue to never cheat, many find a planned cheat is far better than continual bad grazing.

Years ago, I recommended that a female strength athlete who was struggling with some size issues consider the 3-Apple a Day Diet from Tammi Flynn. It's simple: You add an apple to breakfast, lunch and dinner.

A suggested plan from the site *everydiet.org* includes this daily menu—

Breakfast

Apple
Cheese omelet
1 cup cooked oatmeal

Morning Snack

½ cup cottage cheese
½ cup nonfat yogurt

Lunch

Apple
Grilled chicken breast
2 cups steamed broccoli
½ cup brown rice

Afternoon Snack

Cappuccino shake

Dinner

Apple
Grilled salmon
Green salad

The athlete's response was classic: That is waaaay too much food. I had her analyze two days of her typical intake and she discovered, much to her amazement, that the bagels, French fries and pizza she had been eating (and the BEER!) were far more calories than this little recommendation.

The moral of this first part is simple: Most people know what to eat. St. Jean, Ferris and Flynn's ideas are all well within the range of normal. There is no mention of HCG, exotic herbs or excessive measurements of anything. I spent several months categorizing the various low (low carb and low fat are the most common) and high (high fiber, high protein and, yes, even high fat) diets just to get a sense of how things flow through time. I can guarantee that if low-carb diets are popular this year, next year's answer will be high carbs, in some form.

When people see these three recommendations, many walk away from the sensible advice because it is "too much food." It's funny to watch the opposite happen, too. My good friend and partner in a recent training workshop, Dr. Jeff McCombs, has a wonderful approach to dealing with systemic Candida and all the various symptoms that branch out from this condition. One of the things he asks people to give up while dealing with this situation is oranges. Very simply, Jeff asks people starting the regime to stop eating oranges and drinking orange juice. In his practice, people have noted issues with oranges and he advises…for this issue…to avoid them. It's a simple request and Jeff is a gentle man.

Then someone asked me about Dr. McCombs' approach. "I like it! In fact, one of the things that got me thinking was his issue with oranges, I started to…" I never finished the sentence. "What? What's wrong with oranges?" "Oh, nothing, but Jeff has found that having people give up oranges seems to…" Again, I never finished that sentence. "I couldn't do that. No. Not oranges."

This is something I have seen before. If you want adolescent boys to get into an area, put up a sign that says "Restricted." One of my thoughts to increase reading among teens is to put "No Entrance" signs in libraries and have long lists of banned books. If I tell you to not eat oranges for a few months, the only thing most people can think of is eating oranges!

If we tell you NOT to eat certain things, you crave them. If we tell to you eat other things, you don't want them. So, there you have it. We have a barbell issue with most people when it comes to food. The barbell is an excellent way of imagining a graph with highs on both ends and lows in the middle. If I tell you to eat all the vegetable soup and salad you want for the rest of your life, you will find a dozen excuses not to "eat that much." On the other hand, if I tell you to give up a single item, well, then, it's on! We drift back into that middle area of foods like chips and sodas and breads and cereals and graze ourselves up to a nice level of morbid obesity.

All of this reminds me of my little experience with crying when I realized I wouldn't eat again for a week. It is hard to believe that after centuries (millennia!) of struggling to find enough to eat, we now have an emotional response when we are allowed to eat all we want, save for "this."

That might be the beauty of Lent or any other communal fast. For 40 days, you give up this or that and have the support of others marching the same path. Moreover, if done for religious reasons, you can also assume God has a stake in your success. I gave up soda drinks for Lent in the eighth grade and noticed an interesting thing: I never drank them again. If it takes 28 days or 40 days to make a new habit, maybe you should start today.

It's a funny thing about soft drinks. I worked for 54 weeks in a Cheese Factory as part of the night clean-up crew. We had a solvent called Liquid K, which is also the same thing as dishwasher fluid. It makes water wetter. It's also the chemical that keeps many soft drinks from turning into solids on the shelf. It might be worthy of a second thought the next time you take a refreshing break.

The other issue that has arisen in the past few years is the gooization of many foods. I just invented the word, gooization, but you know it. If you go to New York and get a bagel with some cream cheese, some lox, a little onion and some capers, you have an interesting mix of protein, fats and veggies. If you go down to a motel for its free break-fast, you now get chocolate chip bagels or blueberry bagels with spreads that are more sugar than anything else. It's gooey and it's good. Yum. What was once probably a fine snack, the bagel, like many foods, has turned into another sugary treat.

Yes, you know: *Eat like an adult.*

Advice for Everyone, Everywhere, Every Time

I have a standard three-part formula for the past years for most of the people I help.

1. **More protein**
2. **More fiber**
3. **More fish oil**

Protein

I'm amazed to continue to write "more protein" after all these years. I even rediscovered I was the biggest sinner when I took on the challenge of the Velocity Diet. Every few hours, I pounded down a protein shake. I began to notice little things like how good my skin felt and how clear my thoughts were throughout each long day at work. It began to dawn on me that many of my mood swings through the day reflected my diet choices. My strength went up, too, by the way, as I famously broke the state record in the snatch the week after finishing the diet.

It was just a few years ago I realized even though "Eat More Protein" is great diet advice, there's an enormous disconnect. I had a student raise her hand in my weights class to ask, "Where do you get protein?"

I was stunned. Growing up, diet information was part of our health classes. We also discussed not sticking things in your ears, bicycle safety, situational awareness in life and many other things. Sadly, most health classes today focus on sexuality and the diseases related to sex. And, more sadly, I wish I was joking. At best, a student might be shown the food pyramid developed by the Department of Agriculture that emphasizes grains and milk products. By the way, read *The Omnivore's Dilemma* for all you will EVER need to know about corn.

I stood there in that room and realized my student had no idea what this magic protein means for her. She didn't know, at an oddly basic level, how to eat. I asked Robb Wolf, author of *The Paleo Solution,* about this and he told me an interesting thing that still bounces around in my mind. Many people, and perhaps even you, can tell me that Vitamin C prevents scurvy or that lack of Vitamin D can lead to bone issues. But when asked *What is a good breakfast?,* the same person will be at a loss.

It could be the conflicting advice given on television and radio literally every few minutes. Wave after wave of advertising rushes past our eyes and ears urging us to eat or drink this or that. A sugary cereal is part of a good breakfast (!) when you include orange juice, two pieces of toast with butter, some bacon and two eggs. The cartoon characters selling the cereal take up the bulk of the commercial and the balanced-breakfast picture lasts for a second.

It should have been a shock to find that my student, a product of an amazing school system and an elite private high school, couldn't come up with a food that contained protein. This young lady might be well aware that a certain nutrient can do this or that, but to manage a diet, she was lost.

Protein rich foods

> **Meat**
>
> **Fish**
>
> **Eggs**
>
> **Dairy products**
>
> **Legumes (beans and peas)**
>
> **Nuts and seeds**

Notice Tim Ferriss' recommendation to combine protein (meat, fish, eggs) with legumes (beans) to actually gives you a little extra bang for the buck. The upside of this advice is that our friends, the beans and peas, are very high in fiber.

I also include protein powders to this list. An important point: A few years ago, I would not have included powders. When I was growing up, proteins were simply awful: awful tasting, awful digesting and, maybe, awful for you. Soy-based proteins and odd-tasting combinations of this and that were more appropriate for punishment than for human intake. For whatever reasons, modern protein powders actually digest well and don't have that metallic aftertaste of the old flavors.

One caveat about protein powders: Make sure they are low carbohydrate. For a serving size, and this will vary with the size of the little scoop provided, look for probably five grams of carbs or fewer per serving. Often, the extra carbs are simple sugars and most people just don't need that in their diets.

In a bulking program, protein, as its root meaning suggests, stands in the front.

Fiber

If there is an area most people need to rethink in their diets, it is fiber. In the 1960s, the first discussions of fiber and the need for more fiber in the American diet began to be written. With highly processed foods, it was argued, Americans were losing natural sources of fiber and setting themselves up for all kinds of issues later.

Folks, it is "later." Some authorities, like Dr. Scott Connelly of the *Body RX* book, offer that we should consume up to 60 grams of fiber during fat-loss phases of our training. One of my favorite books on the subject, *The F Plan Diet*, has recently been retooled in *F2,* and both books argue for a serious meal-to-meal commitment to fiber.

Everydaydiet.org offers this daily F2 menu—

> **Breakfast**
> Cereal/fruit mix (special recipe) with low-fat milk
> Piece of fresh fruit

> **Lunch**
> Nutty coleslaw
> Fresh fruit

> **Dinner**
> Skinless baked chicken
> Baked potato
> Mixed Salad

> **Drinks**
> Calorie-free drinks, tea and coffee with low-fat milk

The special mix is in the book—it contains a wealth of fiber.

Fiber intake almost has a magical relationship to lean body mass and good health. Certainly, if you are interested, there is a myriad of material both on the internet and in bookstores that will spell this out in more detail than one would ever actually want to know.

Fish oil

Finally, on fish oil: If there is a magic supplement for most people as this is being written, it is fish oil. Recently, well-accomplished strength coach Charles Poliquin of *Charlespoliquin.com* wrote an excellent piece on why fish oils are the most important supplement. In it, he outlined the benefits of fish oil as follows—

Fish oils have been promoted as a potential cure for virtually all diseases. Some members of the medical community have inferred that most ailments can be healed by manipulating the ratios between the EPA and the DHA.

For those of us interested in positively and optimally altering body composition and maximizing our training efforts, fish oils offer 16 possible advantages.

1. Has positive effects on any disease known to man. According to the Natural Medicines Comprehensive Database, fish oils have been shown to have medical applications in the treatment of an extremely wide variety of ailments including hyperlipidemia, hypertriglyceridemia, coronary heart disease, cardiac arrhythmias hypertension, stroke, bipolar disorder, rheumatoid arthritis, psoriasis, atopic dermatitis, ulcerative colitis, Behcet's syndrome and Raynaud's syndrome.

Fish oils are also used orally for weight loss, asthma, cancer, painful menses, lung diseases, hay fever, Crohn's disease, chronic fatigue syndrome, albuminuria associated with diabetic neuropathy, restenosis after angioplasty, miscarriage, pre-eclampsia, preterm labor and intrauterine growth retardation.

Fish oils are used for systemic lupus erythematosus, cystic fibrosis, gingivitis, renal impairment associated with cirrhosis, hyperglycemia associated with type 2 diabetes and claudication. Fish oils are also used to treat attention deficit hyperactivity disorder (ADHD), dyslexia and dyspraxia.

2. Cell membrane health. Eicosapentaenoic acid (EPA) and docosahexaenoic acid (DHA) insure that cell membranes remain healthy. This means the membranes are flexible and contain larger numbers of insulin receptors that are more receptive and responsive to circulating insulin. This results in decreased fat storage in the adipocytes (fat cells).

3. Fish oils turn on the lipolytic genes. That means the genes responsible for burning fat are activated, which means an increased utilization of fat stores from the adipocytes.

4. Fish oils turn off the lipogenic genes. The fat storage genes are turned off.

5. Fish oils diminish C-reactive proteins. This is a newly identified risk factor associated with various inflammatory diseases, including atherosclerosis, angina, coronary heart disease, heart attack, stroke, congestive heart failure and diabetes. The DHA fraction of the fish oil seems to be the one most responsible for the protective effect. DHA also has best ability to reduce blood pressure.

6. Reduced inflammation from physical training. EPA has the greatest effect on reducing inflammation through its downstream metabolites known as resolvins. Resolvins may be the key to the beneficial actions of fish oil in human diseases.

7. Pain management from the reduced inflammation. While fish oils reduce pain and inflammation themselves, they are also displacing other more pro-inflammatory fats out of the cell membranes, providing an additive effect. When people improve the omega-6 to omega-3 ratio, they report a noticeable improvement in pain.

8. Increased focus in training. EPA regulates blood supply to the brain, which is essential in maintaining focus in weight training sessions. DHA is important in brain membranes, memory and cognitive function.

9. Fish oils increase serotonin levels (the happy neurotransmitter). Therefore, fish oils decrease incidence of depression, anxiety, panic attack and reduce carbohydrate cravings.

10. Fish oils improve cardiovascular risk profile. Fish oils lower VLDL, triglycerides, homocysteine and fibrinogen, and increase HDL levels. Combining fish oils with plant sterols will improve lipid levels even more than either alone.

11. Fish oils can also decrease blood pressure by several mechanisms. These include increases in the vasodilatory compound, nitric oxide, reducing vascular inflammation, blocking the constrictive elements in the vascular wall such as the calcium channels reducing blood viscosity, and inhibiting a blood vessel constrictor (thromboxane). Lipoprotein (a) is another CVD predictor that can be lowered by fish oils—a 19% reduction was seen with natural, stable fish oils and just 4% with a highly purified fish oil.

12. Fish oils are a great stress fighter. Supplementation with n-3 fatty acids inhibits the adrenal activation of steroids, aldosterone, epinephrine and norepinephrine (catecholamines) elicited by a mental stress, apparently through effects exerted at the level of the central nervous system. Therefore, under the same amount of stress, one will produce fewer stress hormones if consuming fish oils on a regular basis.

13. Fish oils turn on the carnitine enzymes. These are the enzymes responsible for the burning of body fat.

14. Fish oils mitigate insulin response. This means blood sugar won't rise as quickly and sugar is less likely to go to the fat cells.

15. Fish oils reduce arterial stiffness and increase vasodilation. This benefit, which is good for both heart health and athletic performance, has been shown to take effect in four hours or less.

16. Offers very easy compliance. Taking fish oil on a regular basis is something very easy for people to do. Nearly all obese people are depressed, so for them, because it raises serotonin, taking fish oil could be the first essential step toward a lean healthy body.

You can read the article in full, as well as the continuing commentary, at the following link: *http://www.davedraper.com/url/poliquin.php.*

I have a hard time believing anything else can come close to this list. Fish oil is your one-stop shop of supplements.

Let's start with the bane of most lifters' life in the gym: squats. Years ago at a clinic a young man told me, "Squats hurt my knees." I asked him to demonstrate a squat and responded bluntly, "Squats don't hurt your knees; what YOU are doing hurts your knees." Squats can do more for total mass and body strength than probably all other lifts combined. Doing them wrong can do more damage than probably all the other moves, too.

Any properly executed squat, however, may be a more effective muscle-builder than all other exercises combined. It requires the synchronized recruitment of muscle fibers throughout the body. Because squatting is one of the most natural human movements, like walking or using the remote, it's perfectly safe. And new research shows that squats burn up to three times as many calories as previously thought—this type of leg exercise is a powerful fat-burning tool.

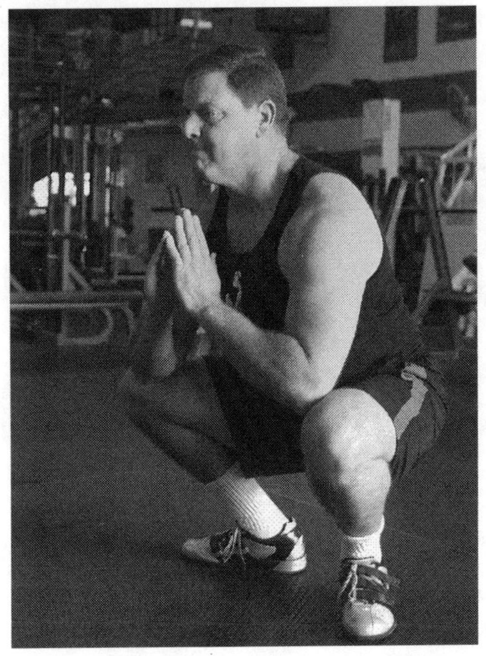

Let's start simple. Find a place where no one is watching and squat down. At the bottom, the deepest you can go, push your knees out with your elbows. Relax…and go a bit deeper. Your feet should be flat on the floor. For the bulk of the population, this small movement—driving your knees out with your elbows—will simplify squatting forever.

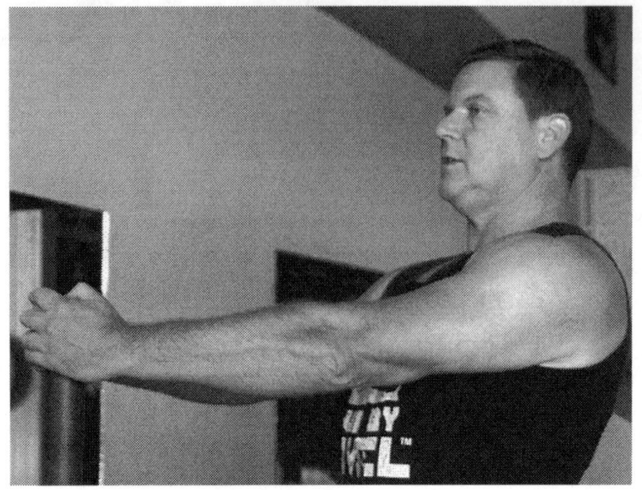

Next, try this little drill: Stand arms-length from a door knob. Grab the handle with both hands and get your chest up. Up? Imagine being on a California beach when a swimsuit model walks by. When I have an athlete do this, immediately, he puffs up the chest, which tightens the lower back and locks the whole upper body. The lats naturally spread a bit and the shoulders come back a little.

Now lower yourself down.

What people discover at this moment is a basic physiological fact: The legs are NOT stuck like stilts under the torso. Rather, the torso is slung between the legs. As you go down, leaning back with arms straight, you will discover one of the true keys of lifting: *You squat between your legs.* You do not fold and unfold like an accordion; you sink between your legs. Don't just sit and read this: Do it!

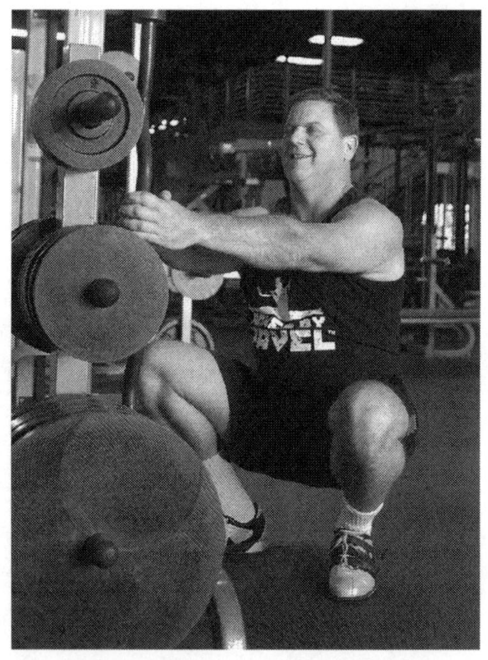

Now you are ready to learn the single best lifting movement of all time: **the goblet squat.** Grab a dumbbell or kettlebell and hold it against your chest. With a kettlebell, hold the horns, but with a dumbbell just hold it vertical by the one end…like you are holding a goblet against your chest. You see, goblet squats.

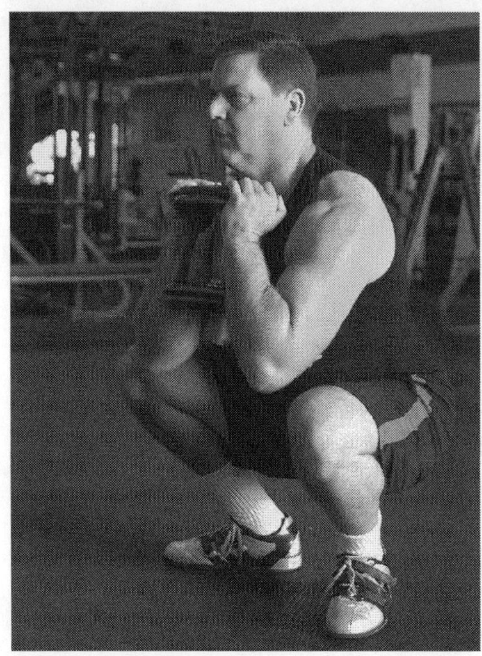 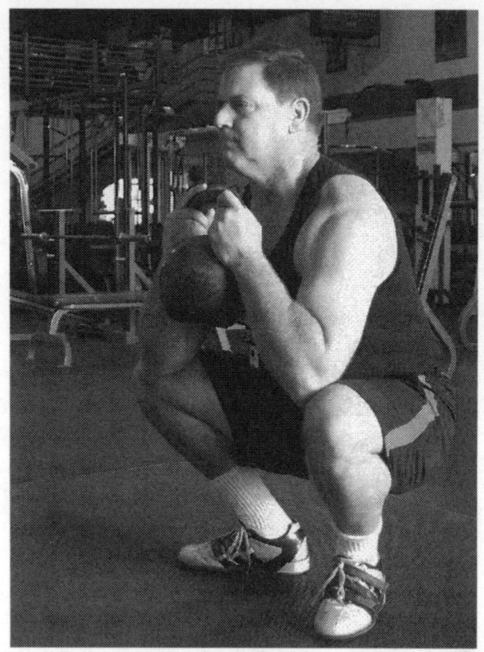

Now with the weight cradled against your chest, squat down with the goal of having your elbows—pointed down because you are cradling the bell—slide past the inside of your knees. It is okay to have the elbows push the knees out as you descend.

There is the million-dollar key to learning movements in the gym: *Let the BODY teach the body what to do.* Listen to this: **Try to stay out of it!** Thinking through a movement often leads to problems; let the elbows glide down by touching the inner knees and good things will happen. The more an athlete thinks, the more the athlete can find ways to screw things up. Don't believe me? Join a basketball team and get into a crucial situation. Shoot a one-and-one with three seconds to go, down by two points…get back to me later if you decided "thinking" was a good idea.

I'm not sure I should tell you this, but I think goblet squats are all the squatting most people need. If the bar hurts in back squats (I won't comment), your wrists hurt in front squat (swallowing my tongue here) and the aerobics instructor has banned you from using the step boxes for your one-legged variations, try the goblet squat. Seriously, once you grab a bell over 100 pounds and do a few sets of 10 in the GS, you might wonder how the toilet got so low the next morning. If you have never squatted before, let me walk you through my "system."

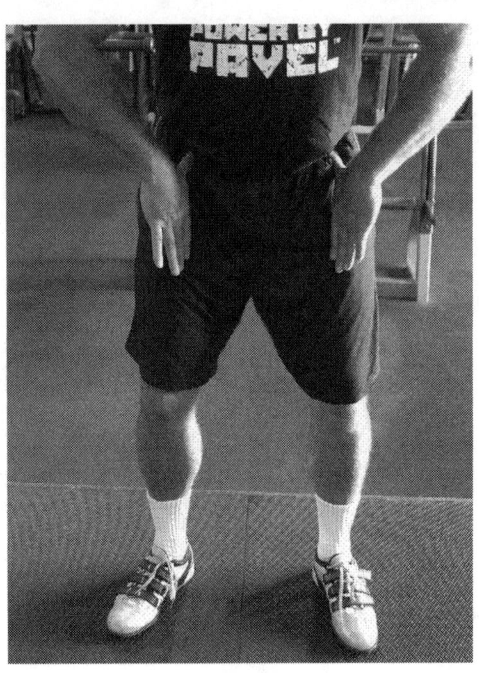

1. Squat with Your Elbows

First, do three consecutive vertical jumps, then look down. This is roughly where you want to place your feet every time you squat. You know, the toes should be out "a little" but most people look down and see the toes magically "out." You don't want to go East and West, but you want some toe-out.

Set your feet and bend your hips and knees to lower your body as far as you can. Then, when you're in your deepest position, push your knees out with your elbows. Try to keep your feet flat on the floor and allow your butt to sink below knee height.

Relax in this position for two or three seconds, then descend a bit deeper and drive your knees out with your elbows once more. For most people, this small elbow maneuver will simplify squatting forever, because it makes us drop the torso between the thighs rather than fold at the waist.

2. Do the Doorknob Drill

You may think of the squat as a lower-body exercise, but proper upper-body alignment is essential. Perfect your posture with this drill. By staying tight through your chest, shoulders and core muscles, you distribute weight more evenly throughout your body. As a result, you'll be able to handle greater loads with less risk of injury.

For review:

Stand an arm's length away from a doorknob and grab the handle with both hands. Set your feet as you did in step one.

Now imagine that you're walking into a bar full of swimsuit models. Your natural reaction will be to immediately lift your chest, which in turn will tighten your lower back. Your latissimus dorsi muscles will naturally spread a bit and your shoulders will move back slightly. I have had dozens of women laugh and tell me that the imagery works for them, too.

Holding the doorknob, keeping your chest up and arms straight, bend your hips and knees to lower your body, and lean back. Then stand up.

3. Now, the Goblet Squat

The goblet squat is named for the way in which you hold the weight—in front of your chest, with your hands cupped. The goblet squat may in fact be the only squat you need in your workout.

Start with a light dumbbell, between 25 and 50 pounds, and hold it vertically by one end. Hug it tight against your chest.

With your elbows pointing down, lower your body into a squat. Allow your elbows to brush past the insides of your knees as you descend. It's okay to push your knees out.

Return to a standing position. Your upper body should hardly move, as if your upper body was in a vertical tube from ceiling to floor. You should feel little movement back and forth and, ideally, none side to side with the upper body if you're using your legs, hips and lower back as a unit.

Don't worry if this isn't perfect the first time. Most people mess up when they think about the move. Just let your elbows glide down by rubbing past your knees, and good things will happen.

The Six-Week Squat 101 Workout

If you are a raw beginner, male, the goal for this is to do a 100-pound goblet squat in just six weeks using this plan. Your upper body stays rigid, so your glutes, quadriceps and hamstrings do most of the heavy lifting. One hundred pounds may not sound all that impressive, but wait till you try it. Once you're able to bang out a few sets of 10 with triple-digit weight, you'll realize the full-body benefits of squats.

Weeks One and Two: Hone your technique. Five days a week, perform two or three sets of five to 20 repetitions of goblet squats. Use a light dumbbell, or even a heavy book.

Week Three: Do squats three days a week, resting for at least a day between sessions. You'll improve your technique and increase strength and muscle endurance.

Day One: Perform a rack walk-up. Grab the lightest dumbbell you can find and do a set of five goblet squats. Return the weight to the rack and grab the next heaviest dumbbell. The exchange should take you no more than 20 seconds. Do another set, then continue moving up the rack until you find a dumbbell that's challenging to lift but still allows perfect technique.

Day Two: Do the reverse of Day One: a rack walk-down. Start with your second-heaviest dumbbell from Day One, and complete a set of five reps. Move down the rack, lifting a lighter weight for each set of five. Aim for a total of 10 to 12 sets, resting for no more than 20 seconds between sets.

Day Three: Combine your workouts from Day One and Day Two. You'll start by moving up in weight, performing sets of five repetitions. When you reach your heaviest weight, work back down the rack. Rest for two days before your next squat workout.

Week Four: Same as Week Three, but perform three reps with each dumbbell, using heavier weights than in your last workout.

Week Five: By now you should feel comfortable performing the goblet squat. You'll focus on building muscle and strength. Again, rest for at least a day between workouts.

Day One: Do two sets of 20 repetitions using a dumbbell that challenges you in the last five reps. Rest for two minutes between sets.

Day Two: Choose a weight that makes it difficult to complete 10 reps. Do three sets of eight reps, resting 60 seconds between sets.

Day Three: Perform a rack walk-up. Do three reps with each weight, and stop when you feel your technique beginning to falter.

Week Six: This week's theme is simple: If you can pick it up, you can squat it.

Day One: Do the regular rack walk-down, performing three reps per set with a heavy weight. Then do it again, this time starting with a slightly heavier dumbbell. Rest for no more than 20 seconds between sets and for 30 seconds between walk-downs.

Day Two: Do a couple of light warm-up sets of goblet squats, then do the rack walk-up twice. Do three reps per set and rest for up to 30 seconds between sets.

Day Three: Do a few easy sets to warm up. Then find the heaviest dumbbell you can lift—aim for three digits—and perform the goblet squat.

The Squat Program

Like just about everything else in this program, there are a few tweaks for the daily squat program. First, there is something you need to know.

You are ONLY going to do high-repetition squats. That means the bar is going to be on your back awhile. If you don't know how to squat, I insist you go through the Six-Week Squat program just outlined. It works. It is better than jamming yourself into the rest of this "stuff" without any orientation. Trust me on this…please, I beg you, if you can't squat, take the six weeks to master it!

Since you are only doing high-repetition squats, you're going to spend a lot of time under the bar. Some of you may complain it hurts your neck or shoulders or whatever. Well, tell someone who cares! Ah, that's not true: If it is a real issue, get Dave Draper's Top Squat attachment for the bar. I used it one time and then purchased one for my home and five for my gym. If you are in so much pain from the bar on the neck or you can't get your arms back far enough (alas), you won't focus on the leg work. It is just one of those things.

Second, I have some strong opinions about the weights you will be using on the bar. The weights on the bar should be what I call "natural weights." If you take a 45-pound plate and pop it on the bar and add another to the other side, that is 135. I don't want any of those fives, tens or two-and-a-half pound plates in this training, just the "natural" 45s, 35s and 25s.

Why? Well, for one thing, when you do a lot of reps, the weights move. They do. Yes, I know there are ways to make them not move, but the little ones like to dance to the end of the bar more than the big ones do. So, we are going to banish the little ones. Next, it also makes it easier to plan and program a routine without having to worry about the small details. And five-pound plates are small details!

If you can't handle the loads, perhaps you need to move to a lighter weight and follow the program exactly. If you simply can't do that, I have to ask if you tried the six-week dumbbell program. If you did, move down to even lighter weights. If you are 135 and below, you might want to try more machine training, as maybe your basic strength levels need some work. If you didn't try the six-week program, well, then do it!

Remember, this program is focused on people who have tried and failed other bulking programs in the past or would like to try an approach that has been very successful. Trust me on this: Having simple numbers in the squat routine is far better than micro-adjustments and percentages. Every second in this program when your brainpower is directed away from the focus of those big sets of squats is a waste of energy. Focus on the squats.

If you are 135 pounds or less, these are the weights you will use—

     45 (the empty bar)

     95

     115

     135

If you are 135 pounds to 185 pounds—the bulk, ahem, of people who have done this program—these are the weights you will use—

    45 (the empty bar)

    95

    115

    135

    185

If you are 185 to 205, you will use these weights—

    45 (the empty bar)

    95

    115

    135

    185

    205

For everyone else, including guys who weigh a "lot" more, these are the weights—

    45 (the empty bar)

    95

    115

    135

    185

    205

    225

I have found little value in doing high-repetition squats over 225 pounds for the people interested in this program. A taller, long-limbed guy who starts getting ugly with a squat over 300 is often heading for an injury quite quickly.

The Miraculous Peanut Butter and Jelly Sandwich

You could have sat me down in 1975 and told me this and I would have shaken my head and walked away. The same could be said for 1985, 1995 and 2005, by the way; I wouldn't have believed you. The following sentence, and I am amazed to say it, is true, for as far as "true" can be for training and nutrition: The peanut butter and jelly sandwich may be the ideal bulking program snack.

Now, raise your hands and ask—

"Isn't tuna better?" "Aren't hard-boiled eggs better?" "Sardines?"

Yes. Yes, to all of your better ideas. I know this is true because I was the guy cracking open hard-boiled eggs every few hours and literally shoveling them down with a healthy washing of water on top. I kept a can opener with me, too, for those delicious raw tuna meals.

Yes, it works. However, if you have tried and failed on a bulking diet before, why not try something that tastes good, delivers a ton of calories and (get ready for it) might be pretty good for you?

Now I'm sure that blended tuna and eggs is "better." Enjoy that for six weeks.

Of course, I recommend high-fiber bread—there are dozens of good options in the grocery stores these days. Also, I would prefer you find a low-sugar jelly or alternative, and look for a "healthy fat" peanut butter. You can even find peanut butter enriched with Omega-3s now. You can get nearly 10 grams of fiber and a healthy hit of protein with a PB&J, and keep the calories between 200 and 500 per sandwich.

Moreover, there is an important point here. It is possible to eat, without wanting to vomit or die, several peanut butter and jelly sandwiches a day. If you have tried to eat massive amounts of less-palatable foods on a bulking program, you will welcome the PB&J snack. Toss in an apple and this whole thing might be too easy to believe. I would be remiss if I didn't add a point given to me by a young lady a few years ago, "Peanut butter and jelly is good for the environment." I have no idea why, but if you need to be Heroically Green while bulking, toss that around when people ask about your diet.

There are other suitable options for snacks, of course, but be sure your options are—

1. **Easily transported**
2. **Easy to consume**
3. **Easy to make**
4. **Something you will actually eat**

Five Additional Hints

1. Stop

One of the most overlooked aspects of muscle-building programs is a four-letter word—**STOP.**

Stop playing basketball. Stop jogging. Stop doing step aerobics class. I swear, if I get one more email that says something like this, I will do something rash—

"Hey, Dan, I'm interested in doing Highland Games. I want to put on some weight, but I have MMA classes three days a week, play in two basketball leagues, and I want to do a marathon. What lifts should I do to put on 60 pounds?"

I tell you, that's not an exaggeration. It's not. Learn to walk slowly. Learn to lie down. Learn to nap. I have argued my whole coaching career that the single hardest thing to do is do add quality lean muscle mass. Now, I didn't say weight—the people with the Big Gulps and doughnuts have bravely shown us that way. I said lean muscle mass.

2. Get Lean, then Gain Mass

One person in a hundred will have the courage to listen to my best piece of advice to prep for a mass-building program: **Lean out first.** My buddy in college who decided to enter an amateur bodybuilding contest lived for a month on nothing but lettuce and dope. Yes, you read that right, and no, don't try it. For his last workouts, his friends had to literally pull him off the floor to do anything. The loads on the bar were far, far below his normal training numbers. But under the lights he looked marvelous.

A funny thing happened the weeks and months after the contest—the guy exploded. It was like he was being inflated. He gained size, in all the right places, seemingly every day. I know there's a scientific explanation for this, but I don't care. I found the same thing happened to me after the Velocity Diet. A week later, I lifted in an open Olympic lifting meet and everyone swore I had put on 10 pounds of muscle when I was actually two pounds lighter. If you have the courage to lean out, try it!

3. Follow the Plan. Complete the Mission.

You need to up the workout intensity. In college, I became "famous," as the local radio and newspapers mention repeatedly, for drinking cold coffee and eating a grapefruit before competing. Two things. First, I didn't normally drink coffee, so I did get a bit of a buzz, and, two, I'd read somewhere that something in the grapefruit made the caffeine work better. There was probably some truth in that, but whatever it takes to get you going, take it!

Ingest whatever you think is appropriate—there are many options at the Biotest store or at the local gas station to give you a buzz. While you're waiting for this to kick in, look at your workout, double-check the numbers and commit to it!

For the rest of your career remember this advice: If I have a million-dollar training idea, it is this—*Write down the plan for your training before you begin.* Try it.

4. Stay Warm to Get Big

I thought Dick Notmeyer was crazy when he told me to stay warm when I was trying to get bigger. He suggested keeping a sweatshirt on at the gym and to wear sweaters and jackets and to not let myself get cold. This is old-school advice, folks, but some of the research on shivering and brown fat might support this idea.

If your body is trying to let you get a little bigger, but you insist on shivering, freezing and shaking, the body is going to shift resources to producing heat. Maybe this is pure fluff, but it's simple enough to try.

Think of it this way. While those 142-pound geeks are walking around in their wife-beater shirts, tribal tats and shaved arms, you can be like that Arnold guy who used to keep an air of mystery about him.

5. When in Doubt, Eat More Protein

Again, do I need to tell you to take more protein? If there was a single great lesson from my experience on the Velocity Diet, it was that I don't get enough protein. I've read many arguments against this, but my experience and my coaching have underscored this simple point. It can be in shakes, post-workout drinks, meat, fish, more eggs or whatever, but get more protein! Please.

Principle-Based Bulking: The Six-Week Approach

The following one day on, two days off workout is the probably the "best" option for our bulking needs. It combines plenty of rest time between workouts, and a recharge the day before each workout. It is not for people who need to do something all the time and every day. Of course, those people often fail on their goals of bulking, too. The other issue with this program is that you need to have a lifting facility that is open seven days a week and you have to commit to training on those days.

If you must, you can work out on this program two days a week. Pick something like Monday/Friday, Tuesday/Saturday or Wednesday/Sunday. Simply slide the program into an additional week before assessing.

If you wish to add another workout or two into the program, and I strongly advise you don't, then do what you want. Just remember it is no longer the program I advise! This is an important point and often missed by people. If you adapt this and this and that, you are no longer doing the prescribed program and you might be sucking the air out of your success.

The one day on, two days off workout assumes that the one day of working out is going to be stressful.

Each training day is followed by two full days of rest, although there is a recommendation for a refresh and recharge workout two days after each training session—the day before the next one.

The six-weeks chart out like the one on the following page.

	Monday	Tuesday	Wednesday	Thursday	Friday	Saturday	Sunday
Week 1	Train **Day 1**	Rest	Re-charge	Train **Day 2**	Rest	Re-charge	Train **Day 3**
Week 2	Rest	Re-charge	Train **Day 4**	Rest	Re-charge	Train **Day 5**	Rest
Week 3	Re-charge	Train **Day 6**	Rest	Re-charge	Train **Day 7**	Rest	Re-charge
Week 4	Train **Day 8**	Rest	Re-charge	Train **Day 9**	Rest	Re-charge	Train **Day 10**
Week 5	Rest	Re-charge	Train **Day 11**	Rest	Re-charge	Train **Day 12**	Rest
Week 6	Re-charge	Train **Day 13**	Rest	Re-charge	Train **Day 14**	Rest	Re-charge
Week 7	**Assess the program**						

Rest

We will start with the simple day, Rest. There are a lot of misconceptions about rest days. I strongly encourage you on the rest days to attempt to do practically nothing in terms of physical work. Avoid playing basketball games, skiing, jogging or running a marathon.

Rest days are ideal for taking care of the business of bulking. This is the day to make extra sandwiches, to prep food. I use this day to soak beans, prepare oatmeal, and even host a "practice Thanksgiving" with everything, including the stuffing. This is the day you want to shop, cook, prep, soak and store food. You want to wake up in the mornings knowing what you are going to eat, when and where.

I highly encourage a duffle bag or small carryall to take food and water and fish oil capsules with you everywhere. Remember, this is not a lifetime habit, just something you need to do for six weeks. You cannot get behind on meals. It may seem odd at first, taking a loaf of bread, a jar of peanut butter, some jelly and sandwich bags and making 12 or more sandwiches. Yet if I were to argue for only one key, it is this: *You must have most of your meals ready to go on the days you are training.*

Don't lose any mental or emotional focus packing and sorting food on the training days. The rest day only refers to resting from the weightroom; **it is not a rest from the commitment to bulking up.** This is exactly where people fail: They train hard for two or three sessions, then toss away all the momentum on the rest days. You must work as hard on the rest days—taking care of rest day business—as you do on the training days. Oddly, I find the smarter and harder I work on the rest days, the more intense become my training days.

The Bulker's Shopping List

The Eat Like an Adult List

* Poultry
* Sausage
* Bacon
* Fish
* Shellfish, if you're not allergic to it
* Canned tuna
* Salmon (in the can or fresh—the king of grilled foods!)
* Eggs (buy them in the five-dozen containers)
* Heavy cream, for coffee, if you use it
* Real butter, if you use it
* Cheese, (okay for some people, not for others)
* Salad greens—everything you can eat raw
* Vegetables (I use frozen bags of veggies and microwave them as a side dish)
* Lemons and limes to sweeten drinks and squeeze on fish and salads
* Herbs and spices
* Olive oil
* The best in-season fruit

Our Super-secret Bulking Foods

High-fiber bread
Low-sugar peanut butter—with Omega-3 if you can find it
Low-sugar jelly (do your best)
Beans (black, pinto, white)
Supplements
Fish oil
Quality creatine powder
An excellent non-soy protein powder

When you get home, make your sandwiches, organize a few meals and generally get ahead of the curve here.

Recharge

Recharge is a term Dan Martin and I have been using in our discussions concerning how to refresh and recover from really hard training after, shall we say, a certain age. What most people discover after about age 30 is that a little bit of the hair of the dog that bit you goes a long way in helping you recover for the next day's workout.

I get sore when I squat. In hindsight, I have always gotten sore when I squat. No real surprise there, but when I try to walk up a flight of stairs after a hard squat workout, the last thing I want to do is more squats.

But that is the answer! A few light squatting moves seems to "grease the groove," as Pavel says, and gets things moving again. My Recharge Workout is something that looks somewhat like a mobility workout and somewhat like a weight workout. I don't worry about sets or reps or load, I just move around.

It doesn't have to be much. When I work with people in groups, I often get requests for the name of this exercise or that exercise, but some of the exercises are simply stuff like Ed's Really Good Leg Stretch. Don't make it too complex. Think about a squat, a walk, a pull, a push and a hinging movement, and stretches for anything that is stiff, sore or needs love.

I have had success with doing a few sets of goblet squats, some yoga cobras and downward dogs, a couple of easy sets of swings and some presses. It doesn't have to be hard or long or organized. Just move around for 10 to 20 minutes. Yes, it is that simple.

If you have something like a TRX and a kettlebell, move through a basic workout, but keep the times shorter and the intensity very low. If you have no tools on hand, try some yoga or a just go for a nice walk. Some parks have some fitness stations, walk and do some of the movements.

Are you getting the idea? Move!

Record Your Progress

If I could suggest ONE thing for lifelong success in sport, finances or anything really, it would be to **keep a journal or diary.** This will give you a window on how you progress to your goals. I have been keeping a journal since 1971 and it is by far the best tool I have for tracking how I achieve my goals. For example, I tend to do better when I am early. "Early" means a lot of different things to me—it would including showing up early, sending registrations in early and the like, but it also means I seem to thrive when I take care of business early…proactive, if you will. How do I know this? My journals record this time after time. What makes you succeed? Find out by keeping track of things.

The cheapest pen is better than the finest memory, it has been said, but in lifting, our memories fade with each second off the platform. Don't trust "what you think" you did in reps with 225…write it down!

You'll find a six-week logbook beginning on page 120.

These changes and additions—tweaks—are strategically placed. There's a reason I put them in each spot in the program. Don't get gung-ho and add everything at once. Do the program as written.

Week One

Week One has three workouts and no tweaks. That's not really true. I do expect you to begin experimenting with three meals and multiple snacks each day. Hopefully, the workouts will "insist" that you go to bed earlier.

Successful bulkers learn quickly to carry a backpack with a couple of peanut butter and jelly sandwiches and some apples. Actually, the apple is good advice, as peanut-butter breath gets old really fast. I tend to buy a two-liter bottle of something, pour the contents out or give it away, and continually refill it with tap water throughout the day. Two or three snacks several times a day is going to help you bulk up certainly, but it will also keep you glued on the process of gaining mass. Every time you sling that backpack over your shoulder, let it be a reminder of what you are trying to accomplish over the next six weeks. Don't ignore this simple little trick!

Week Two

I suggest you begin this the night of Training Day Three.

Of all the things I have ever tried, this is the most universal of the small tricks that work for most people. Honestly, I have never had this technique fail me or anyone I have ever worked with in training.

It is very simple: Drink a protein shake before going to bed. Usually the recommended serving size is two scoops, so use this as your guide: This is a two-scoop shake. Now, raise your hands and ask, "What do you mean 'before you go to bed'?" Simply, drink it within an hour or two of when you think you will be asleep. Please don't read much more than that into this. I don't want to know the details about how long it is before when you go to bed and when you go to sleep. Thank you.

There are at least a two good reasons why this works. First, many of us "starve" from dinner to breakfast. It can be up to a 12-hour fast. Knocking down a low-carb protein drink won't have much of a hit on your blood sugar, but it will give the body something to work with overnight.

And, as fellow RKC Tim Ferriss notes, it might just make your next day better—

> *Morning fatigue and headache isn't just from sleep debt or poor sleep. Low blood sugar following overnight fasting is often a contributing factor. Just prior to bed, have a small snack such as a few sticks of celery with almond butter, a mandarin orange and five to eight almonds or plain low-fat (not fat-free) yogurt and an apple. Ever wonder how you can sleep eight to ten hours and feel tired? This is part of the explanation. Make a pre-bed snack part of your nutritional program.*

~ From Tim Ferriss' blog

Tim, a bestselling author, is, along with A. J. Jacobs, someone who really makes me rethink just about everything.

Assess this every morning. Does it work for you? *Working* means some movement upward on the scale and perhaps better sleep and general recovery. If it does work, keep this little trick in your permanent training regime. Obviously, if it is working, continue doing this through the whole bulking program, too.

If it isn't, well, I have no experience with this, so let's have you consider the quality of your protein, the stresses in the rest of your life and perhaps reconsider moving through the rest of the program for now. It just might not be the right time for you to work on bulking.

Week Three

A couple of years ago, I had a great chance, literally hours, to talk with Dr. Tom Fahey. You think you don't know Tom, but, well, you probably do. His textbook is the standard for college exercise majors; he is the editor of a major muscle magazine and is a world-class masters discus thrower. In this conversation, he simplified all the research of all the studies of all the sports with this statement—

> *"Well, once you get to a certain level, you just need to get your deadlift and bench press higher, as nothing helps as much as absolute strength for an elite athlete."*

I love the simplicity of that.

For nutrition, he summed the whole thing—

> *"This is interesting, Dan. If you take about 10 grams of protein—not much, really— before you train, there is research, solid stuff, that says it goes right into the muscles— just as we had always hoped it would."*

Tom went on to explain in it in maddening detail and you must trust me when I tell you I understood practically nothing after the key point.

But, what a key point! So, before you train, drink a one-scoop protein drink. Between warm-ups and the general training, you have time before the more "puke-inducing" parts of our program.

This is an amazingly simple little addition. It does take some planning—remember to pack a scoop of protein in your backpack and something to add water to mix it in. There are plenty of shake blenders available at every single store I seem to walk into lately. Splurge. Get one.

Week Four

Add creatine. Listen, creatine has its own Wikipedia section now. The early warnings when the product first became famous have been largely disproven. Not too many years ago, a parent showed up to school with her son's container of creatine and asked, "Is this really anabolic steroids like my sister told me?"

No. Now, does creatine work as miraculously for everyone as some ads promise? Well, no. In fact, it just makes me a little goofy in the belly. However, when my athletes pack on a lot of weight quickly and their lifts go up quickly by just adding a small dose (look how small those serving spoons are in the containers), I can't ignore it.

Just add the smallest amount each day, usually five grams. If you have no problems with it, keep taking it. It used to be argued we need a two-week period to load creatine, but we don't see that very often anymore. Take the creatine in the morning with your breakfast and mix it any way you like. Here's the deal: If it works for you, take the least you need to take, but take it for a long time.

Notice how each week we are adding a sensible, low-level addition to our program. If it works for you, we will continue doing this. For some people, some suggestions don't work and, honestly, no one can tell you why some things work sometimes and don't at other times. Keep these ideas in your training quiver, though. Maybe another time you can come back and these will accelerate your success.

Week Five

This little addition is so obvious, I have a hard time holding my athletes back from trying this too soon: Add a two-scoop protein shake at rising, first thing in the morning. Some have reported this has an effect on breakfast by changing how they feel about eating. It is interesting because after a discussion, usually we find the breakfast choices actually become better after this shake. Instead of reaching for just anything, the protein seems to curb the intense hunger. Dr. Bob Arnot argued the same point in his 1998 book, *Dr. Bob Arnot's Revolutionary Weight Control Program* by having his dieters drink a full glass of skim milk to allow some proactive meal choices in the next few hours after rising.

This is also a great thing to do far beyond a mass-building program. This is the kind of thing you can do for a number of goals, including fat loss, mass building's weird little brother.

It's simple. It works.

Week Six

Of all the tweaks, this final one is the trick that is the most individual of all. So, let's try it with our last two workouts and give it a look. Simply, after finishing your workout, have a one-scoop protein drink. I would suggest it be at least half an hour after squatting, and it would be best to be closer to an hour. With cool-down and recovery, and let's be honest, that set of 50 is going to take a while to recover from, you might have little interest in anything for a while. When I did this program, I couldn't trust riding my motorcycle because I couldn't trust my feet to change gears or brake for a while. Yes, it is that tough.

If you like this one, keep using it. There is some discussion about the validity of post-workout drinks. Some argue it is the single finest thing ever in the field of body-building. Others maintain that it suppresses growth hormone. I have never been one for extremes, but I can attest that it worked for me as an adult to drive my squat and clean & jerk through the roof. So, again, let's give it a few workouts and see.

Week Seven: Assess

There are little dozens, maybe hundreds of programs you can follow. My good friend Dan Martin often calls me Mister 91, because many programs get you in shape in two weeks, two months or 90 days. What about the next day?

That's where my strengths lie. Ongoing success in lifting and body compositions (and life!) is the skill of assessing what works *and* what doesn't work for an individual.

One warning: At the end of the six weeks, stop with high-rep squats for a while. One interesting thing I noticed after high reps is that my attitude towards leg work was forever changed. After doing 50 reps with 225, it doesn't seem like much to do a set of five with that weight as a warm-up. Moreover, it is hard to convince oneself that a leg machine is "just the same" as squatting after spending eternity under a high-rep squat set.

I suggest exploring complexes after these six weeks. Try some of the variations you'll find beginning on page 106. Also, return to some "traditional" training movements—it's completely up to you to define that idea. I prefer things like military presses, deadlifts and front squats (as well as the Olympics lifts), but each of us have our own needs.

Hopefully, you are now eating like an adult! That alone will carry you to many of your future goals. I suggest backing off the peanut butter and jelly sandwiches when you are not doing the high-rep squats. As you honestly look over the six weeks, what parts worked? Did one tweak do better than all of the others for you? It might not be a bad idea to order them up from…

Best to Worst

__________________ **Protein before bed**

__________________ **Protein before the workout**

__________________ **Creatine**

__________________ **Protein upon arising in the morning**

__________________ **Protein after the workout**

This won't be scientific, but take a minute to do this. Oddly, the one you rank at five might be the one to explore either by trying again after NOT doing it for a while or to ask around or use the internet and find those who had success with it. Maybe the amounts you used were too low, which is great and an easy fix, or it could be something else. Obviously, keep numbers one and two close to your chest. Those are your personal "secret" weapons.

When you get to the workout log sheets, you'll understand how important your note-taking is. There's space to keep track of how well these tweaks work, or don't work, and, as always, I highly encourage good note-taking throughout the program.

Also, take some time to think through the workouts. Yes, they're simple—

Four lifts (really only two)

One unchanging complex

High-rep squats

If you made progress, how complex (in the other sense of the word) does your training need to be?

How you measure success, too, is very important. I have received reports of this program putting on three pounds a week! But, as I have often written, what do these pounds on the scale mean?

Others have been amazed by the amount of arm growth with no arm work. That's not true: You do plenty of arm work, but no direct arm work. It's the secret of true size, if you want to know the truth.

Okay, get your hat on and put on your game face. Let's cheer and hoot and pound the walls—it's time to work out. Beyond a simple warm-up and cool-down, the workout will be in three phases.

Upper-body strength work

Complexes

High-repetition squats

One of the biggest issues most people who have failed bulking programs in the past have is that they really get too hung up on doing lots of things and miss the keys to muscle gain. First, you must get stronger. Second, you have to spend some time under a load.

There is nothing else, really, in the weightroom.

The problem with lower-body work for many guys is that the Olympic bar sits on the ground at a height determined a long time ago. And that is fine. However, a quick look at the full height of most Olympic lifters and elite powerlifters will tell you an interesting fact: The weightlifting sports favor the shorter athlete. Even the space between the collars limits taller guys—my "perfect" grip for the snatch is actually wider than where I can hold. Something as simple as deadlifting might be quite fun and exciting for someone five feet tall, but a brutal lower-back lift for an NBA center.

Moreover, I once had a brilliant insight while spotting a guy who played professional basketball. As he descended with the bar to go into the deep squat, he kept going and going and going. Tall guys move the bar a lot farther on barbell lifts than "normal" people. In addition, guys who grow doing just "anything" are not normal either.

This weightlifting program is designed to work with the issues that seem particular to people who find it hard to gain lean body mass.

The Workout Template

General Warm-up

With the literally thousands of warm-up ideas, programs and DVDs available to a trainer today, I don't even know where to begin. Generally, something is better than nothing, but I would suggest doing the following, though feel free to add or subtract anything you like.

1. Get the blood flowing and heat up a bit. Don't go overboard here, but take a few minutes, not more than five, and do something that gets you going. For most big guys, I always recommend an exercise bicycle since many of

these guys have enough joint issues already. Bike riding is fine, or walking or whatever, but just get a little warm and don't ride too far away. A slow run, some arm swinging and some easy movements are fine, too. And, to be honest, sometimes the weather does more to warm you up than anything you can do in the gym.

2. From some good advice from Mike Boyle, I now spend a few minutes on the foam roller. These are very inexpensive and I just roll out my middle back (crack-crack-crack), my IT bands on the outer thighs, my hamstrings and my hips. It takes about two minutes at most.

3. Mike has lately been suggesting static stretching. Static stretching fell out of favor a while ago, but I like targeting tight areas of my body. Almost always, I find my hip flexors, hamstrings and upper back need a few minutes of relaxing into the stretch.

4. Because our workouts start with the upper body, there isn't a lot of need for much else, but I have found that a few swings, a couple of goblet squats and a few strides (a few sprints that I describe as "start off slow and taper off," just some easy gliding sprints at maybe three-fourths exertion to really top off the effort.

Upper-body Strength

Bench Press

Those of you who have read my long rants about how most people waste their time in the gym just bench pressing might be shocked to see this as our first lift. This is an appetizer for the program, the main dish is coming later. In addition, it is hard to argue that any other upper-body movement can handle the amount of weight on the bar that a bench press allows. The other great lift, the overhead press, will be addressed in a minute, so relax.

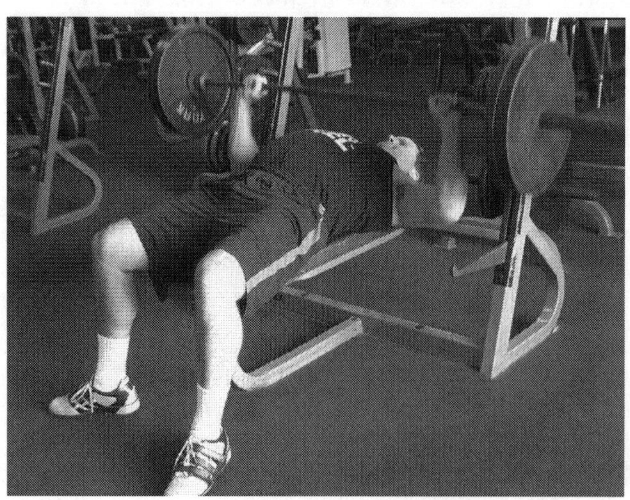

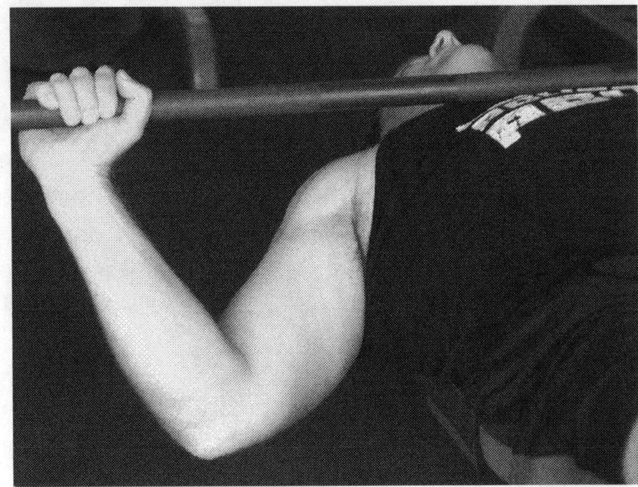

The biggest issue for most people with the bench press is hand position. Often guys will come in the gym, put their hands next to the knurling and lift from there. This is almost universally wrong. The elbows must be "underneath" the wrists in the bench press.

The hand is not above the elbow.

I have had many students watch their peers lift and look for this and they come away amazed at how inefficient their teammates are lifting. (Then, of course, I note that they are doing the exact same thing.) It is well worth your time to take a few minutes to master a grip that will allow you to lift more weight more efficiently.

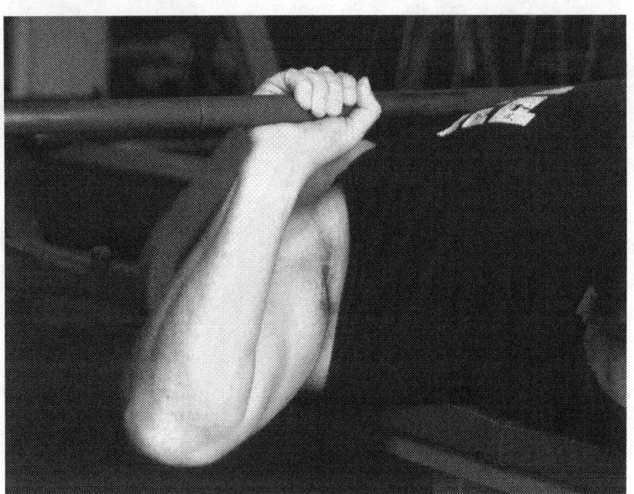

The hand is not in line with the elbow.

In addition, you must have some serious spotters. Now, generally, I wouldn't allow this, but if you can't get quality spotters and you have a machine available, well, then, do it. Just don't tell me. I made amazing progress using the old Universal Bench Press machine, but it too has its limits.

There are plenty of resources to improve your bench. It is worth your time and energy to explore them.

Bat Wings

Today's typical workouts ignore the rhomboids. Developing these muscles in the middle of your upper back will balance your workout and help you stand taller. Moreover, most guys struggling to gain lean body mass also seem to have posture issues that lead to soft tissue problems that lead to long-term issues. Let's fix it now.

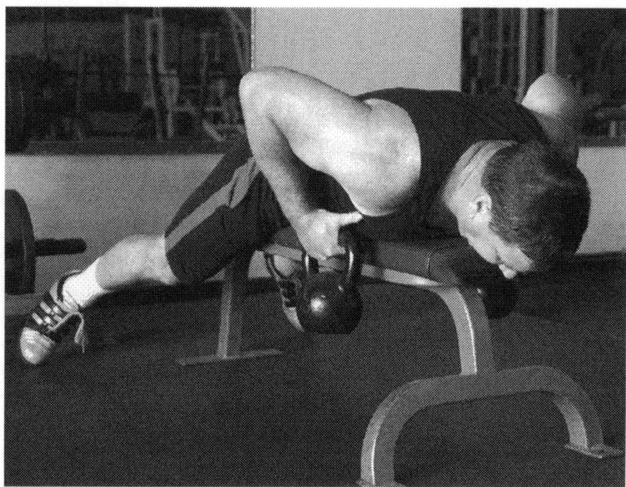

Grab a heavy pair of kettlebells or dumbbells and lie facedown on a bench, resting the weights on the floor. Pull the weights up toward your rib cage, squeezing your shoulder blades together at the top for a second. From a bird's-eye view, your torso should resemble bat wings.

This movement is slight; the weights should move up and down only about six inches. The higher you pull, the harder you should squeeze your shoulder blades together. Perform four or five sets of five repetitions. The repetitions are small, something akin to an isometric squeeze.

One-arm Presses

If I had to pick the single best lift to teach the athlete to provide lean body mass, I would choose the one-arm press. What does it teach? Rooting. Being one piece. Locking down. It also works a massive number of muscles, and the learning curve is straight up. You can learn the one-arm press in seconds and master it in just a few workouts.

Any Russian Kettlebell Certified trainer (RKC—visit *dragondoor.com* for more information) can show you the basics in seconds. Really, it is simple, but I do prefer that you keep an eye on your foot placement. I often do this lift with one foot in the air, just to get a sense of the whole body reacting to the load. It is an interesting little experiment.

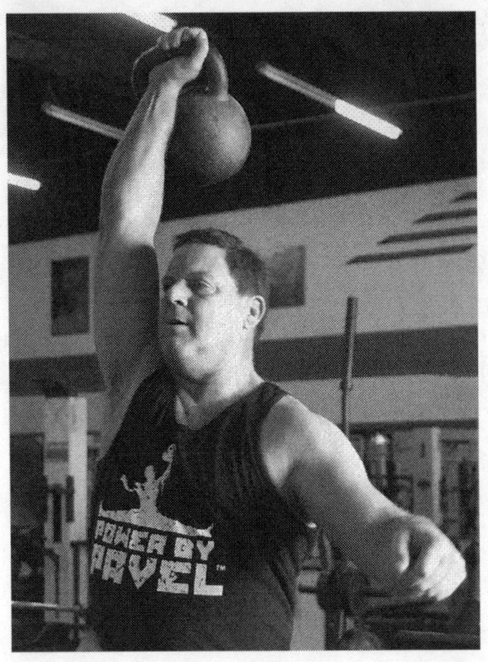

For most workouts, keep your feet tighter than shoulder-width, occasionally even do them heel to heel. As for the movement, be sure to start low (I always touch my thumb on my pectoral to make sure I am in deep enough), and then progress to a total elbow lockout. Don't lead with the trap by shrugging. I like to squeeze my lat to start the movement. If this is too complex, that is my fault. Take a bell, press it overhead. There!

Bird Dog

You will know this one. Or, you should. Get down on your hands and knees. Raise one arm to parallel. Point the arm out straight in front and extend the opposite leg to the rear. Hold it. Repeat to the opposite side.

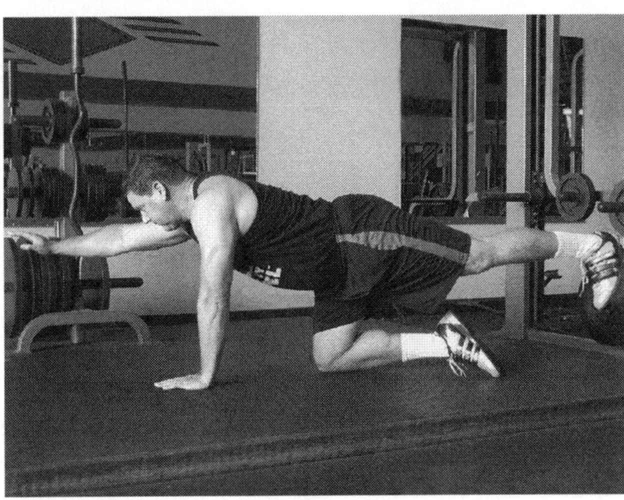

Yes, it isn't much, but it is a great abdominal exercise without crushing your back or burning up too much energy. A bulking period is NOT the time to do a million ab moves. Never, actually, is the time to do a million ab moves.

These four movements are the core of the upper-body strength program. Don't dismiss it as "too little." You have just begun the training day.

Complexes!

For years, I have introduced complexes to my athletes at times when I thought we needed a bit more muscle mass, and when we had nothing too important coming up. I had been exposed to complexes almost from my first days lifting and I wrote a very popular article on them a few years ago. The key point of the article was this—

My definition of a complex is simple. A complex is a series of lifts back to back where you finish the reps of one lift before moving on to the next. The barbell only leaves your hands or touches the floor after all of the lifts are completed. Although you can do them with barbells, dumbbells or kettlebells, I argue to only use barbells. Certainly, there's great value in the other tools, but for getting athletes bigger, I like to use the heavier bar.

The key to organizing a complex is to make sure the bar passes over your head in some kind of logical manner. In other words, if you do rows followed by back squats, how did the bar get there? I try to have the bar pass backwards over the head after a few lifts, but only pass forward again once.

So, when you try these (it's probably best to use a broomstick first), note that it'll save you some effort if you think about the exercise transitions before you go too heavy.

For our six-week assault on bulking, we will only do one complex. There are several reasons. First, it helps to master the combination of movements. I can whip up a new complex in a manner of minutes and that is great if you are in love with variations. Sadly, in my experience the guys with the most variations in their training are usually also the weakest and skinniest.

Second, this complex has a nice mix of pushing, pulling, squatting and bending with just enough rest between to allow some recovery. Some…not much!

Finally, complexes are, well, complex. I don't want you putting the bar down and trying to remember how to do this or that. I want you to stress and strain for those last seconds.

You'll find a section of my favorite complexes beginning on page 109, and you can download a printable pdf off my website, *danjohn.net,* to put on the floor in front of you during the complexes.

Now, recall my definition. A complex is a series of lifts back to back where you finish the reps of one lift before moving on to the next. The barbell only leaves your hands or touches the floor after all of the lifts are completed.

> **Row**
> **Clean**
> **Front squat**
> **Military press**
> **Back squat**
> **Good morning**

If the workout calls for eight repetitions, you need to do eight rows, followed by eight cleans, then eight front squats and so on. Do NOT load up the bar the first few times through—trust me, this is a bad idea.

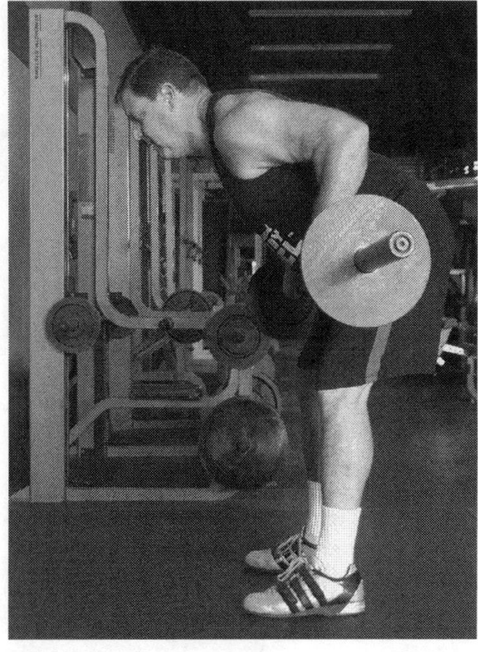

Bentover barbell row

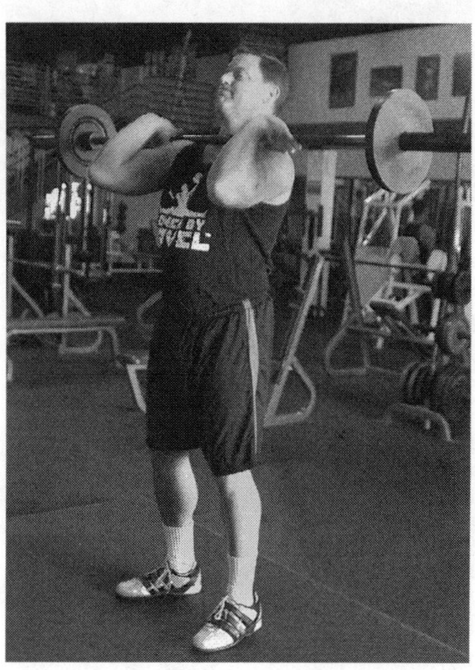

Top of the barbell clean

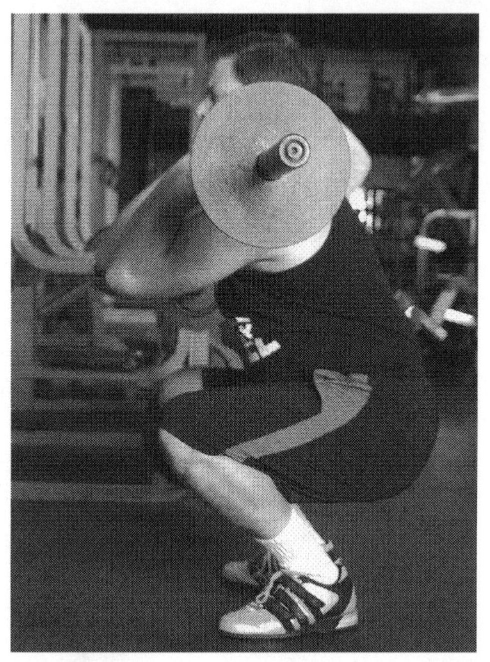

Front squat

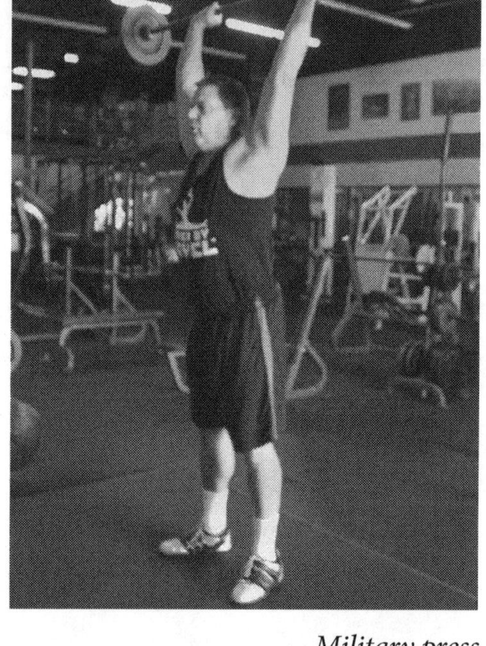

Military press

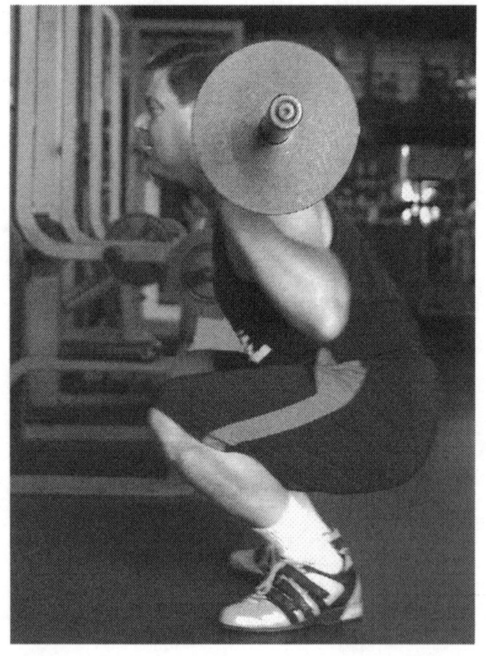

Back squat

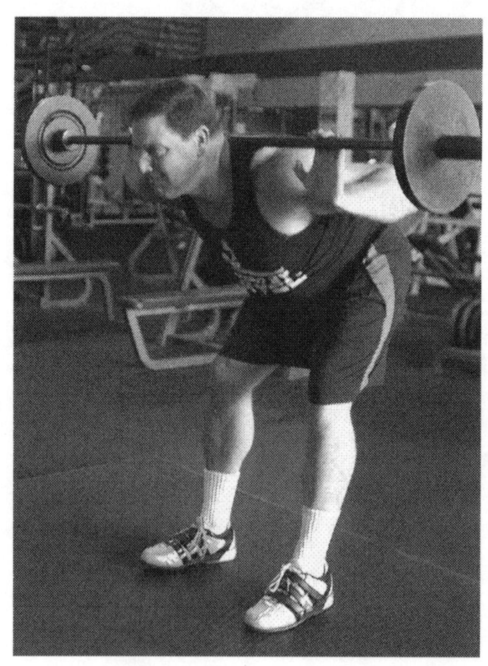

Good morning

High-repetition Back Squats

When I post my workouts online, one of the basic criticisms I receive is "they are too easy" or the "weights are too light." Yet when I work hands-on with real people with lean body mass goals, they universally note that the weights and load are realistic.

So, we back squat with reasonable weights for a lot of reps and grow.

I could type up a bunch of mischief and let you suffer, but I would rather you have a bit of confidence and make the lifts. A couple of things about the back squat—

- Always walk up to the bar, shoulder it and step back to clear the racks.
- You only need to step back with one foot, then the other. Don't go for a walk.
- Be sure to keep your lower back tight, suck in a big gulp of air and make a bold chest.
- Go deep. Really, that's the whole key. Make me proud.
- Get all the reps. Please. If you don't know how to squat, follow the six-week program in this book and learn. If you think you know how to squat but this or that hurts…you don't know how to squat!

The General Warm-up

Warming up is both the most over- and under-complicated aspect of training. I have trained well with no warm-ups and also followed complex dynamic movements coupled with fairly advanced drills. Both work! Let's do the simple things we can do to get started—

1. Five minutes of gentle moving. Get the blood flowing.
2. Foam rolling (middle back, IT bands, hamstrings and hip flexors)
3. Static stretches for hip flexors, hamstrings, upper back and hot spots
4. Some easy swings, goblet squats and a few strides

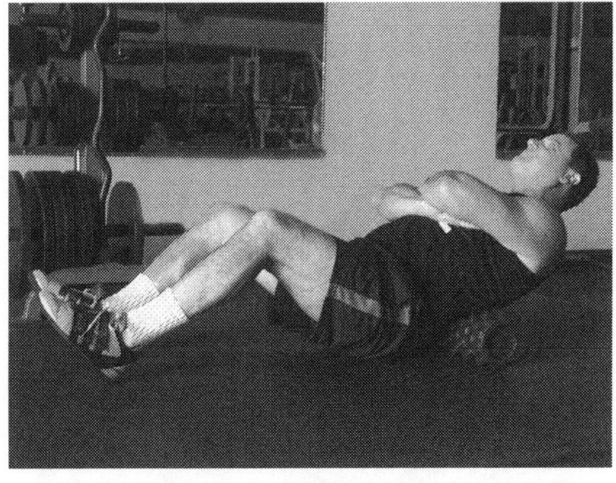

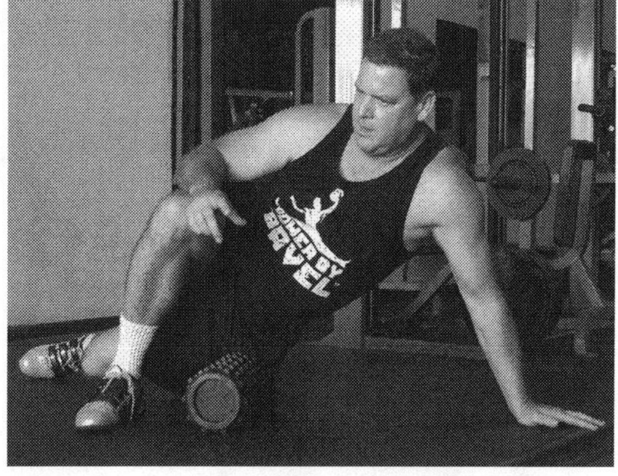

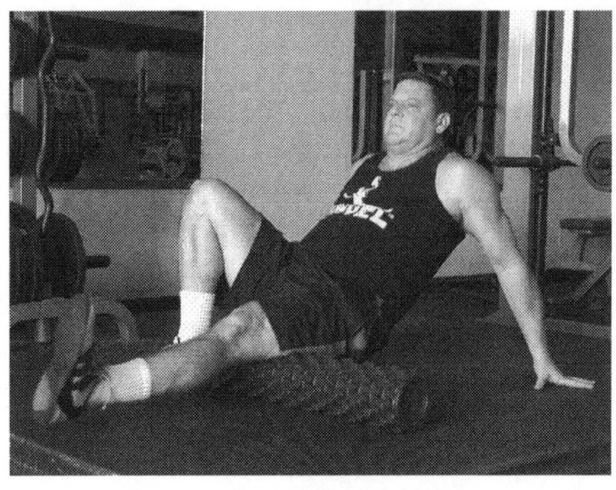

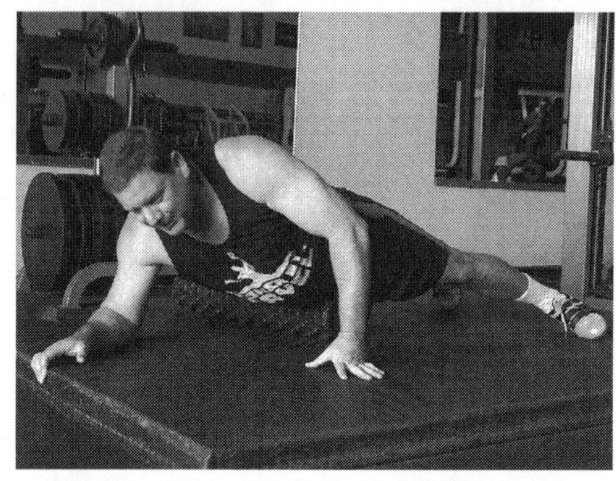

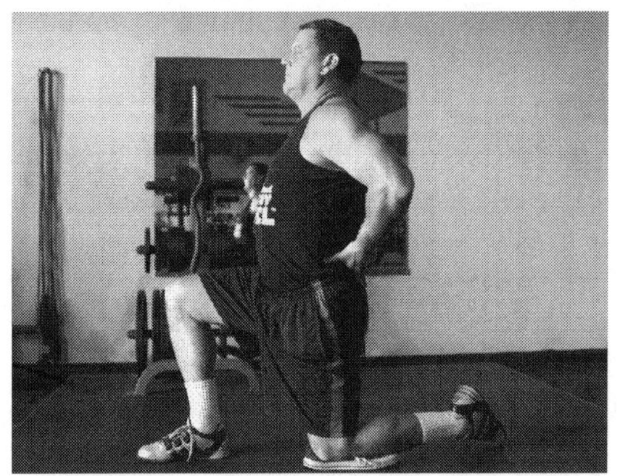

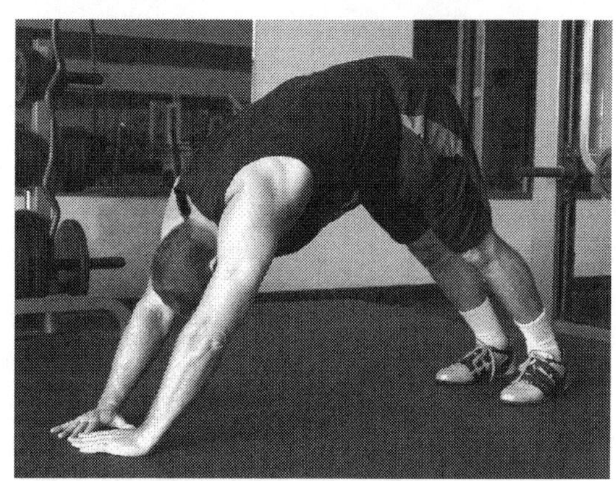

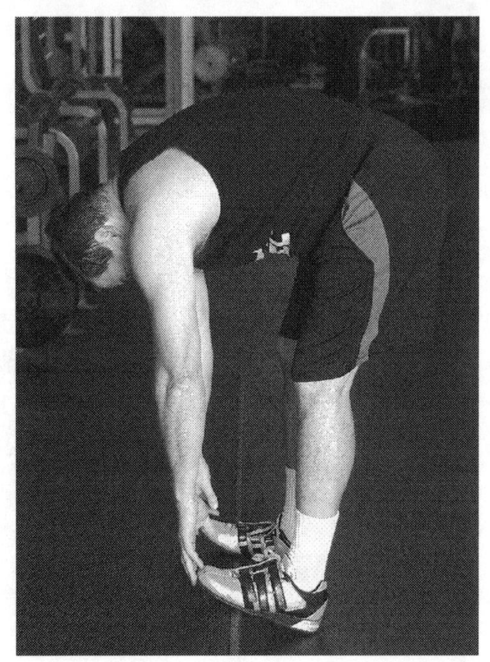

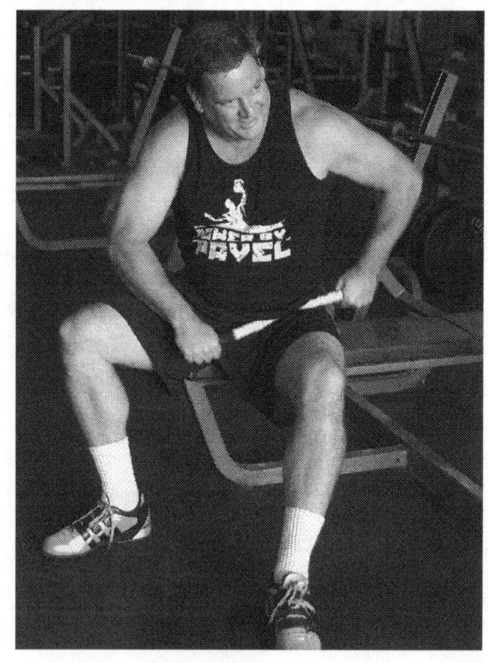

Cool -down

After one of my workouts, I laid down on the cement in front of my house. When I recovered, I looked up to see my dog sitting next to me with a very concerned look. Another time, I finished a strongman event and collapsed. My wife was reassured with, "Don't worry, we only thought he was dead for a second or two."

I have had "cool-downs" that consisted of me sitting on a bench for a long time trying to figure out how to drive home. I have also had long, lovely cool-downs of sauna, steam and whirlpool.

The point of all of this is simple: *Have some kind of transition from the gym back to life.*

It is a good time, during the cool-down, to do more mobility work and maybe even work some kinks out. I have worked on technical things during a cool-down and found it effective for me to unwind from the load. Do something for a few minutes to make sure your heart has slowed down and your brain can make two connected thoughts. Then, go eat and rest. We will see you again in a few days.

I'll ask you to record your training weights, and we'll build on these during the course of the program. This may look confusing as you're reading the text, but once you get to the weightroom, you can use the workout log at the end of this workbook. Referring back to the numbers from the previous workouts will be easy once you put the program into action.

The actual workouts come next.

General warm-up

1. Five minutes of gentle moving. Get the blood flowing.
2. Foam rolling (middle back, IT bands, hamstrings and hip flexors)
3. Static stretches for hip flexors, hamstrings, upper back and hot spots
4. Some easy swings, goblet squats and a few strides

Bench press

Please take a few minutes to warm up with appropriate light weights to prepare yourself for the heavier movements. Today is a simple break-in workout. Do a set of five repetitions with an easy weight, then add more weight, do another set of five. I want to find a weight you can do a comfortable set of five. With wise weight selections, this should take about five or six sets.

5 sets of 5, ascending weights

With the top "comfortable" weight, perform an additional set of five.

Write down this final weight: _________________.
You will be using this weight quite a bit for a few weeks.

Bat wings

Today, just orientate yourself with the movement. I want you to try several different dumbbells or kettlebells to find the right weight. Hint: It might be lighter than you think.

Hold the weight in at the armpits for a 10-second count for two sets.

Write down this weight: _________________.
This will be your base weight.

One-arm presses

If you have a rack of dumbbells or a series of kettlebells, I want you to walk up the weights, start with your weaker arm and do two to five repetitions per weight. Don't try to kill yourself. Match this with your stronger arm. Repeat on both the weaker and stronger arms.

Write down the heaviest weight you used today: _________________.
This will be the weight that will begin Day Two.

Bird dog

Practice the movement a few times. Do both sides and master the movement. Move your knees closer together over time.

Complex

A complex is a series of lifts back to back where you finish the reps of one lift before moving on to the next. The barbell only leaves your hands or touches the floor after all of the lifts are completed.

1. Row for three repetitions
2. Clean for three repetitions
3. Front squat for three repetitions
4. Military press for three repetitions
5. Back squat for three repetitions
6. Good morning for three repetitions

With an empty barbell, perform the entire complex one time through to familiarize yourself with the movements. If you can, add a little weight (65–95 pounds is actually about right for most men. Do two more additional complexes, all the movements done back to back to back for three repetitions. If you can keep adding weight, do so.

High-repetition back squats

One set of 30 with 95 pounds

If you are under 135 pounds, just use the empty bar and thank me later.

Cool-down

Take some time transitioning back to the real world. This is also a nice time to do anything you think you might need to do. I use this time for my corrective exercises for any injuries or issues that have appeared over the past season.

General warm-up

1. Five minutes of gentle moving. Get the blood flowing.
2. Foam rolling (middle back, IT bands, hamstrings and hip flexors)
3. Static stretches for hip flexors, hamstrings, upper back and hot spots
4. Some easy swings, goblet squats and a few strides

Bench press

Please take a few minutes to warm up with appropriate light weights and prepare yourself for the heavier movements.

With the weight from last workout, perform the following—

Do two repetitions, rest a little.

Do three repetitions, rest a little.

Do five repetitions, rest.

This is the *2—3—5 Workout.* It will be the base of most of your training. Do the "set" of *2—3—5* twice.

Bat wings

Do 10 five-second holds with the weight used on Day One.

One-arm presses

Take a few easy warm-ups with lighter weights, then progress to your training weight. Begin with the weaker arm and do *2—3—5.* Switch to the stronger arm and do another "set" of *2—3—5.* Repeat this for a total of two sets.

Bird dog

Practice the movement a few times. Do both sides and master the movement. Move your knees closer together over time.

Complex

Repeating: A complex is a series of lifts back to back where you finish the reps of one lift before moving on to the next. The barbell only leaves your hands or touches the floor after all of the lifts are completed.

I repeat this because people invariably get it wrong.

1. Row for three repetitions
2. Clean for three repetitions
3. Front squat for three repetitions
4. Military press for three repetitions
5. Back squat for three repetitions
6. Good morning for three repetitions

Today, do the complex five times. Do not keep adding weight after the third complex. The weight you are using for sets three, four and five will be your target for the next workout.

High-repetition back squats

Two sets of 30 with 95 pounds

If you are under 135 pounds, just use the empty bar for the first set and add a pair of 10s (65 pounds total) for the second set. Yes, this breaks the rules of big plates, but go with me on this.

Cool-down

Take some time transitioning back to the real world. This is also a nice time to do anything you think you might need to do. I use this time for my corrective exercises for any injuries or issues that have appeared over the past season.

Program reminder

This is your last workout with no tweaking. Get ready for some excitement next week.

General warm-up

1. Five minutes of gentle moving. Get the blood flowing.
2. Foam rolling (middle back, IT bands, hamstrings and hip flexors)
3. Static stretches for hip flexors, hamstrings, upper back and hot spots
4. Some easy swings, goblet squats and a few strides

Bench press

Please take a few minutes to warm up with appropriate light weights and prepare your-self for the heavier movements.

With the weight from last workout, perform three "sets" of *2—3—5*. If you complete all the repetitions, please add a reasonable amount of weight for the next workout.

2—3—5 weight = _________________, three rounds

Goal weight for next workout = _________________

Bat wings

Do 10 five-second holds with the weight from Day One.

One-arm presses

Take a few easy warm-ups with lighter weights, then progress to your training weight. Begin with the weaker arm and do *2—3—5*. Switch to the stronger arm and do another *2—3—5*. Repeat this for a total of three sets.

2—3—5 weight = _________________, three rounds

Next time, go up to _________________

Bird dog

Practice the movement a few times. Do both sides and master the movement. Move your knees closer together over time.

Complex

Again: A complex is a series of lifts back to back where you finish the reps of one lift before moving on to the next. The barbell only leaves your hands or touches the floor after all of the lifts are completed.

1. Row for five repetitions
2. Clean for five repetitions
3. Front squat for five repetitions
4. Military press for five repetitions
5. Back squat for five repetitions
6. Good morning for five repetitions

Remember to use the weight from the last sets of Day Two.

Today, do two complexes.

High-repetition back squats

One set of 30 with 95 pounds, then one set of 30 with 115 pounds

If you are under 135 pounds, just use the empty bar for the first set and add 10s (65 pounds total) for the second set.

Cool-down

Take some time transitioning back to the real world. This is also a nice time to do anything you think you might need to do. I use this time for my corrective exercises for any injuries or issues that have appeared over the past season.

Program reminder

Tweak—You should be on your third day of the late-night protein drink. Ideally, you have been waking up refreshed. Some have told me soreness is diminished after this regime. If it is working, **KEEP DOING IT**

General warm-up

1. Five minutes of gentle moving. Get the blood flowing.
2. Foam rolling (middle back, IT bands, hamstrings and hip flexors)
3. Static stretches for hip flexors, hamstrings, upper back and hot spots
4. Some easy swings, goblet squats and a few strides

Bench press

Please take a few minutes to warm up with appropriate light weights and prepare yourself for the heavier movements.

Use your new goal weight today. Do two sets of *2—3—5,* then **take your old weight** and do as many safe repetitions (with a spotter) as you can do up to 10 reps.

2 x 2—3—5 weight: _______________________

Reps with original weight: _______________________

Bat wings

Do five 10-second holds with the weight from Day One. Consider going up next week.

One-arm presses

Take a few easy warm-ups with lighter weights, then progress to your training weight.

Begin with the weaker arm and do *2—3—5.*

Switch to the stronger arm and do *2—3—5.* Repeat this for a total of two sets.

2 x 2—3—5 weight:_______________________

Bird dog

Practice the movement a few times. Do both sides and master the movement. Move your knees closer together over time.

Complex

Not again! Yep: A complex is a series of lifts back to back where you finish the reps of one lift before moving on to the next. The barbell only leaves your hands or touches the floor after all of the lifts are completed.

1. Row for five repetitions
2. Clean for five repetitions
3. Front squat for five repetitions
4. Military press for five repetitions
5. Back squat for five repetitions
6. Good morning for five repetitions

Remember to use the weight from the last sets of Day Two, the same weight you handled last time. Today, we do three sets of this complex.

High-repetition back squats

Three sets of 25 with 115 pounds

If you are under 135 pounds, just use the empty bar for the first set and add 10s (65 pounds total) for the second and third set. Today ends the "fun."

Cool-down

Take some time transitioning back to the real world. This is also a nice time to do anything you think you might need to do. I use this time for my corrective exercises for any injuries or issues that have appeared over the past season.

Program Reminder

Tweak—There are only two workouts this week, but a lot of additional protein. This is an important week to track moods and size gains.

General warm-up

1. Five minutes of gentle moving. Get the blood flowing.
2. Foam rolling (middle back, IT bands, hamstrings and hip flexors)
3. Static stretches for hip flexors, hamstrings, upper back and hot spots
4. Some easy swings, goblet squats and a few strides

Bench press

Please take a few minutes to warm up with appropriate light weights and prepare yourself for the heavier movements.

Keep using **your new goal weight**. Do three sets of *2—3—5*.

> **2—3—5 weight:** _________________, **three sets**

Bat wings

Do five 5-second holds with a heavier weight. If it is a miserable failure, go back down. If not, really try to squeeze those shoulder blades together.

One-arm presses

Take a few easy warm-ups with lighter weights, then progress to your training weight.

Begin with the weaker arm and do *2—3—5*.

Switch to the stronger arm and do *2—3—5*.

Repeat this for a total of three sets.

> **2—3—5 weight:** _________________, **three sets**

Bird dog

Practice the movement a few times. Do both sides and master the movement. Move your knees closer together over time.

Complex

No, seriously? A complex is a series of lifts back to back where you finish the reps of one lift before moving on to the next. The barbell only leaves your hands or touches the floor after all of the lifts are completed.

1. Row for five repetitions
2. Clean for five repetitions
3. Front squat for five repetitions
4. Military press for five repetitions
5. Back squat for five repetitions
6. Good morning for five repetitions

Remember to use the weight from the last sets of Day Two, the same weight you handled last time. Today, we continue to do three sets of this complex.

High-repetition back squats

If you are 135 pounds or less, these are the weights you will use—

45 (the empty bar) x 30

45 (the empty bar) x 30

95 x 25

If you are 135 pounds to 185 pounds (most of people who have done this program), these are the weights you will use—

45 x 5

95 x 30

115 x 30

135 x 15

If you are 185 to 205, you will use these weights—

95 x 30

115 x 30

135 x 30

For everyone else, including guys who weigh a "lot" more, these are the weights—

     95 x 30

     115 x 30

     135 x 30

Cool-down

Take some time transitioning back to the real world. This is also a nice time to do anything you think you might need to do. I use this time for my corrective exercises for any injuries or issues that have appeared over the past season.

Program reminder

Tweak—Again there are only two workouts, but you have really gone up on protein intake. Be sure to take one scoop before training.

General warm-up

1. Five minutes of gentle moving. Get the blood flowing.
2. Foam rolling (middle back, IT bands, hamstrings and hip flexors)
3. Static stretches for hip flexors, hamstrings, upper back and hot spots
4. Some easy swings, goblet squats and a few strides

Bench press

Please take a few minutes to warm up with appropriate light weights and prepare yourself for the heavier movements.

Keep using **your new goal** weight today. Today, the first "set" is *2—3—5—10,* as many as **up to 10.**

Record the reps: ___________________

Then, two more sets of *2—3—5.*

Bat wings

Do five 5-second holds with a heavier weight. If it is a miserable failure, go back down. If not, really try to squeeze those shoulder blades together.

One-arm presses

Take a few easy warm-ups with lighter weights, then progress to your training weight. Try to stay with the heavier weights.

Begin with the weaker arm and do *2—3—5.*

Switch to the stronger arm and do *2—3—5.*

Repeat this for a total of three sets. This is our standard one-arm press workout.

2—3—5 weight: ___________________, **three sets**

Bird dog

Practice the movement a few times. Do both sides and master the movement. Move your knees closer together over time.

Complex

Seriously: A complex is a series of lifts back to back where you finish the reps of one lift before moving on to the next. The barbell only leaves your hands or touches the floor after all of the lifts are completed.

1. Row for five repetitions
2. Clean for five repetitions
3. Front squat for five repetitions
4. Military press for five repetitions
5. Back squat for five repetitions
6. Good mornings for five repetitions

We're back to five sets. If you need to go lighter on the first and last sets, that's okay.

High-repetition back squats

Here we begin our *To Fifty* squat workouts. *To Fifty* workouts are simply this: You are going to **do 50 squats TOTAL**. If you can, do one set to 50, or break it up any way you want. Stop immediately if your technique sours, rest and start again.

The goal is to do fewer total sets every session. Don't stop on a predetermined rep like 5 or 10…the goal is to get all 50 reps.

If you are 135 pounds or less, these are the weights you will use—

45 (the empty bar) x 10

45 (the empty bar) x 10

95 to fifty

If you are 135 to 185 pounds, these are the weights you will use—

45 x 5

95 x 10

115 x 10

135 to fifty

If you are 185 to 205, you will use these weights—

>   95 x 10
>
>   115 x 10
>
>   135 to fifty

For everyone else, including guys who weigh a "lot" more, these are the weights—

>   95 x 10
>
>   115 x 10
>
>   135 to fifty

Cool-down

Take some time transitioning back to the real world. This is also a nice time to do anything you think you might need to do. I use this time for my corrective exercises for any injuries or issues that have appeared over the past season.

Program reminder

Be sure to take one scoop of protein before training.

General warm-up

1. Five minutes of gentle moving. Get the blood flowing.
2. Foam rolling (middle back, IT bands, hamstrings and hip flexors)
3. Static stretches for hip flexors, hamstrings, upper back and hot spots
4. Some easy swings, goblet squats and a few strides

Bench press

Please take a few minutes to warm up with appropriate light weights and prepare your-self for the heavier movements.

Max Day: Today's single goal is to get a maximum double. We want TWO REPS with as much weight as you can do. Get a good spotter and make sure you get two clean reps…no help, no bouncing and no cheating.

    Put your max double here: _________________

Bat wings

Do five 10-second holds with your usual weight. Please, for me, try to squeeze those shoulder blades together.

One-arm presses

Take a few easy warm-ups with lighter weights, then progress to your training weight.

Begin with the weaker arm and do *2—3—5*.

Switch to the stronger arm and do *2—3—5*.

Repeat this for a total of "just" two sets.

    2—3—5 weight: _________________**, two sets**

Bird dog

Practice the movement a few times. Do both sides and master the movement. Move your knees closer together over time.

Complex

Right! A complex is a series of lifts back to back where you finish the reps of one lift before moving on to the next lift. The barbell only leaves your hands or touches the floor after all of the lifts are completed.

1. Row for five repetitions
2. Clean for five repetitions
3. Front squat for five repetitions
4. Military press for five repetitions
5. Back squat for five repetitions
6. Good mornings for five repetitions

Just do three sets today, but move the weight up every set.

High-repetition back squats

If you are 135 pounds or less, these are the weights you will use—

45 (the empty bar) x 10

45 (the empty bar) x 10

95 x 10

115 x 5

115 x 5

115 x 5

135 x 5

If you are 135 to 185 pounds, these are the weights you will use—

45 x 5

95 x 10

115 x 10

135 x 10

185 x 5

185 x 5

185 X 5

If you are 185 to 205, you will use these weights—

     95 x 10

     115 x 10

     135 x 10

     185 x 10

     205 x 5

     205 x 5

     205 x 5

For everyone else, including guys who weigh a "lot" more, these are the weights—

     115 x 10

     135 x 10

     185 x 10

     205 x 5

     205 x 5

     225 x 5

     225 x 5

Cool-down

Take some time transitioning back to the real world. This is also a nice time to do anything you think you might need to do. I use this time for my corrective exercises for any injuries or issues that have appeared over the past season.

This is the toughest week of the program. Survive it by following the supplemental tweaks that work for you.

Good luck!

Program reminder

Tweak—This week we are adding five grams of creatine to the daily diet. Be sure to keep up with the other protein supplementation ideas, too. There are three workouts this week, so don't allow your nutrition let you down.

General warm-up

1. Five minutes of gentle moving. Get the blood flowing.
2. Foam rolling (middle back, IT bands, hamstrings and hip flexors)
3. Static stretches for hip flexors, hamstrings, upper back and hot spots
4. Some easy swings, goblet squats and a few strides

Bench press

Please take a few minutes to warm up with appropriate light weights and prepare yourself for the heavier movements.

Today, just add plates until you are **20 pounds under your max double from last time.** With a good spotter, do five doubles with this weight.

Bat wings

Do five 10-second holds with your normal weight, but maybe you can experiment with a heavier weight during at least one of the sets.

One-arm presses

Take a few easy warm-ups with lighter weights, then progress to your training weight. Try to stay with the heavier weights.

Begin with the weaker arm and do *2—3—5*.

Switch to the stronger arm and do *2—3—5*.

Repeat this for a total of "just" two sets.

2—3—5 weight: ________________, two sets

Bird dog

Practice the movement a few times. Do both sides and master the movement. Move your knees closer together over time.

Complex

Yes, you've got it! A complex is a series of lifts back to back where you finish the reps of one lift before moving on to the next. The barbell only leaves your hands or touches the floor after all of the lifts are completed.

1. Row for two repetitions
2. Clean for two repetitions
3. Front squat for two repetitions
4. Military press for two repetitions
5. Back squat for two repetitions
6. Good mornings for two repetitions

This is probably my favorite way to do complexes. Add weight every time, for a total of five rounds. Most people find the military press to be the limiting lift, so use that movement as the gauge for adding weight.

High-repetition back squats

Reminder: *To Fifty* workouts—**do 50 Squats TOTAL.** If you can, do one set to 50, or break it up any way you want. Stop immediately if your technique sours, rest and start again. The goal is to do fewer total sets every session. Don't stop on a predetermined rep number…the goal is simply to get all 50 reps.

If you are 135 pounds or less, these are the weights you will use—

45 (the empty bar) x 10

45 (the empty bar) x 10

95 x 10

115 to fifty

If you are 135 to 185 pounds, these are the weights you will use:

45 x 5

135 x 10

185 x to fifty

If you are 185 to 205, use these weights—

> 95 x 10
>
> 135 x 5
>
> 185 x 3
>
> 205 to fifty

For everyone else, including guys who weigh a "lot" more, these are the weights—

> 135 x 10
>
> 185 x 2–3
>
> 205 x 2–3
>
> 225 x to fifty

Cool-down

Take some time transitioning back to the real world. This is also a nice time to do anything you think you might need to do. I use this time for my corrective exercises for any injuries or issues that have appeared over the past season.

Program reminder

Tweak: This week we've added five grams of creatine daily. Be sure to keep up with the other protein supplementation ideas, too. You've got three workouts this week, and can't allow your nutrition to let you down.

General warm-up

1.   Five minutes of gentle moving. Get the blood flowing.
2.   Foam rolling (middle back, IT bands, hamstrings and hip flexors)
3.   Static stretches for hip flexors, hamstrings, upper back and hot spots
4.   Some easy swings, goblet squats and a few strides

Bench press

Please take a few minutes to warm up with appropriate light weights and prepare yourself for the heavier movements.

Today, add plates until you are **20 pounds under your max double from last time**. With a good spotter, do five triples with this weight.

Bat wings

Do five 10-second holds with your normal weight, or you can move up as long as you can truly hold the shoulder blades together.

One-arm presses

Take a few easy warm-ups with lighter weights, then progress to your training weight. Try to stay with the heavier weights.

Begin with the weaker arm and do *2—3—5*.

Switch to the stronger arm and do *2—3—5*.

Repeat this for a total of three sets.

2—3—5 weight: _________________, three sets

Bird dog

Practice the movement a few times. Do both sides and master the movement. Move your knees closer together over time.

Complex

A complex is a series of lifts back to back where you finish the reps of one lift before moving on to the next. The barbell only leaves your hands or touches the floor after all of the lifts are completed.

1. Row for two repetitions
2. Clean for two repetitions
3. Front squat for two repetitions
4. Military press for two repetitions
5. Back squat for two repetitions
7. Good mornings for two repetitions

We pick up on this same workout from last time. Just do three heavy sets with the weight you finished with last time, if appropriate.

High-repetition back squats

If you are 135 pounds or less, these are the weights you will use—

45 (the empty bar) x 10

45 (the empty bar) x 10

95 x 10

115 x 5

135 x 5

135 x 5

135 x "as many" up to 20

If you are 135 to 185 pounds, these are the weights you will use—

45 x 5

95 x 10

135 x 10

185 x 5

185 x 5

185 x "as many" up to 20

If you are 185 to 205, use these weights—

       95 x 10

       135 x 10

       185 x 10

       205 x 5

       205 x "as many" up to 20

For everyone else, including guys who weigh a "lot" more, these are the weights—

       135 x 10

       185 x 10

       205 x 5

       225 x 5

       225 x "as many" up to 20

Cool-down

Take some time transitioning back to the real world. This is also a nice time to do anything you think you might need to do. I use this time for my corrective exercises for any injuries or issues that have appeared over the past season.

Program reminder

This week you've added the five grams of daily creatine. Be sure to keep up with the other protein supplementation ideas, too. There are three workouts this week, so don't let your nutrition fail you.

General warm-up

1. Five minutes of gentle moving. Get the blood flowing.
2. Foam rolling (middle back, IT bands, hamstrings and hip flexors)
3. Static stretches for hip flexors, hamstrings, upper back and hot spots
4. Some easy swings, goblet squats and a few strides

Bench Press

Please take a few minutes to warm up with appropriate light weights and prepare yourself for the heavier movements.

Using the weight from the last two workouts, get two sets of *2—3—5*.

Bat wings

Do five 10-second holds using a heavier weight.

One-arm presses

Take a few easy warm-ups with lighter weights, then progress to your training weight. Try to stay with the heavier weights.

Begin with the weaker arm and do *2—3—5*.

Switch to the stronger arm and do *2—3—5*.

Repeat this for a total of "just" two sets.

2—3—5 weight: __________________, two sets

Bird dog

Practice the movement a few times. Do both sides and master the movement. Move your knees closer together over time.

Complex

Just in case you don't have it by now: A complex is a series of lifts back to back where you finish the reps of one lift before moving on to the next. The barbell only leaves your hands or touches the floor after all of the lifts are completed.

1. Row for two repetitions
2. Clean for two repetitions
3. Front squat for two repetitions
4. Military press for two repetitions
5. Back squat for two repetitions
6. Good mornings for two repetitions

Using the same heavy weight from last time, do FIVE sets.

High-repetition back squats

We'll be going to fifty again. You should be getting better at the "to fifty" part, taking fewer sets—less rest—to get there. Remember, the goal is 50 reps in a single set.

If you are 135 pounds or less, these are the weights you will use—

45 (the empty bar) x 10

45 (the empty bar) x 10

95 x 10

135 to fifty

If you are 135 pounds to 185 pounds, these are the weights you will use—

45 x 5

135 x 5

135 x 10

185 x to fifty

If you are 185 to 205, use these weights—

95 x 10

135 x 5

185 x 10

205 to fifty

For everyone else, including guys who weigh a "lot" more, these are the weights—

     135 x 10

     185 x 2–3

     205 x 10

     225 x to fifty

Cool-down

Take some time transitioning back to the real world. This is also a nice time to do anything you think you might need to do. I use this time for my corrective exercises for any injuries or issues that have appeared over the past season.

Program reminder

Tweaks—If you are following the tweaks exactly, today—beyond meals and snacks—you will have five scoops of protein and some creatine. Let's make some progress!

General warm-up

1. Five minutes of gentle moving. Get the blood flowing.
2. Foam rolling (middle back, IT bands, hamstrings and hip flexors)
3. Static stretches for hip flexors, hamstrings, upper back and hot spots
4. Some easy swings, goblet squats and a few strides

Bench press

Please take a few minutes to warm up with appropriate light weights and prepare yourself for the heavier movements.

Today, we will once again strive for a max double. With a good spotter, go as heavy as possible for two repetitions.

Write your max double here: _________________

Bat Wings

Do five 10-second holds using a heavier weight.

One-arm presses

Take a few easy warm-ups with lighter weights, then progress to your training weight. Try to stay with the heavier weights.

Begin with the weaker arm and do *2—3—5*.

Switch to the stronger arm and do *2—3—5*.

Repeat this for a total of two sets.

2—3—5 weight: _________________, **two sets**

Bird dog

Practice the movement a few times. Do both sides and master the movement. Move your knees closer together over time.

Complex

Yes! I'm writing it again! A complex is a series of lifts back to back where you finish the reps of one lift before moving on to the next. The barbell only leaves your hands or touches the floor after all of the lifts are completed.

1. Row for five repetitions
2. Clean for five repetitions
3. Front squat for five repetitions
4. Military press for five repetitions
5. Back squat for five repetitions
6. Good mornings for five repetitions

Start with a lighter weight on the first set and then try to match last workout's weight on the last sets. Do three total sets.

High-repetition back squats

Note: For all weights, your goal is to strive for as many reps on the first set of the "to fifty" segment.

Write the rep number from the first set of the "to fifty" here: ________________

If you are 135 pounds or less, these are the weights you will use—

45 (the empty bar) x 10

45 (the empty bar) x 10

95 x 10

135 to fifty

If you are 135 pounds to 185 pounds, these are the weights you will use—

45 x 5

135 x 5

135 x 10

185 x to fifty

If you are 185 to 205, you will use these weights—

> 95 x 10
> 135 x 5
> 185 x 10
> 205 to fifty

For everyone else, including guys who weigh a "lot" more, use—

> 135 x 10
>
> 185 x 2–3
>
> 205 x 10
>
> 225 x to fifty

Cool-down

Take some time transitioning back to the real world. This is also a nice time to do any-thing you think you might need to do. I use this time for my corrective exercises for any injuries or issues that have appeared over the past season.

Program reminder

If you are following the tweaks exactly, today—beyond meals and snacks—you will have five scoops of protein and some creatine. Let's make some progress!

General warm-up

1. Five minutes of gentle moving. Get the blood flowing.
2. Foam rolling (middle back, IT bands, hamstrings and hip flexors)
3. Static stretches for hip flexors, hamstrings, upper back and hot spots
4. Some easy swings, goblet squats and a few strides

Bench press

Please take a few minutes to warm up with appropriate light weights and prepare yourself for the heavier movements.

Take 20 pounds off your max double and do five sets of doubles today.

5 x 2 with ___________________

Bat wings

Do five 5- to 10-second holds using a heavier weight.

One-arm presses

Take a few easy warm-ups with lighter weights, then progress to your training weight. Try to stay with the heavier weights.

Begin with the weaker arm and do *2—3—5*.

Switch to the stronger arm and do *2—3—5*.

Repeat this for a total of three sets.

2—3—5 weight: ___________________**, three sets**

Bird dog

Practice the movement a few times. Do both sides and master the movement. Move your knees closer together over time.

Complex

I know you know this. A complex is a series of lifts back to back where you finish the reps of one lift before moving on to the next lift. The barbell only leaves your hands or touches the floor after all of the lifts are completed.

1. Row for three repetitions
2. Clean for three repetitions
3. Front squat for three repetitions
4. Military press for three repetitions
5. Back squat for three repetitions
6. Good mornings for three repetitions

Using the same heaviest weight from last time, do three sets.

High-repetition back squats

Today with the "to fifty" segment, we try to get one set of 50 with the workout weight.

Write the number from the first set here: _______________

If you are 135 pounds or less, these are the weights you will use—

45 (the empty bar) x 10

45 (the empty bar) x 10

95 x 10

115 to fifty

If you are 135 to 185 pounds, these are the weights you will use—

45 x 5

135 x 5

135 x 10

135 x to fifty

If you are 185 to 205, you will use these weights—

95 x 10

135 x 5

185 x to fifty

For everyone else, including guys who weigh a "lot" more, use—

>   135 x 10
>
>   185 x 2–3
>
>   205 x to fifty

Cool-down

Take some time transitioning back to the real world. This is also a nice time to do anything you think you might need to do. I use this time for my corrective exercises for any injuries or issues that have appeared over the past season.

Program reminder

Tweaks—Take protein before **AND** after this workout.

General warm-up

1. Five minutes of gentle moving. Get the blood flowing.
2. Foam rolling (middle back, IT bands, hamstrings and hip flexors)
3. Static stretches for hip flexors, hamstrings, upper back and hot spots
4. Some easy swings, goblet squats and a few strides

Bench press

Please take a few minutes to warm up with appropriate light weights and prepare yourself for the heavier movements.

Today, add plates until you are 20 pounds under your max double from last time. With a good spotter, do five triples with this weight.

5 x 3 with ________________

Bat wings

Do five 10-second holds with your normal weight.

One-arm presses

Take a few easy warm-ups with lighter weights, then progress to your training weight. Try to stay with the heavier weights.

Begin with the weaker arm and do *2—3—5*.

Switch to the stronger arm and do *2—3—5*.

Repeat this for a total of three sets.

2—3—5 weight: ________________ **, three sets**

Bird dog

Practice the movement a few times. Do both sides and master the movement. Move your knees closer together over time.

Complex

Right! A complex is a series of lifts back to back where you finish the reps of one lift before moving on to the next. The barbell only leaves your hands or touches the floor after all of the lifts are completed.

1. Row for two repetitions
2. Clean for two repetitions
3. Front squat for two repetitions
4. Military press for two repetitions
5. Back squat for two repetitions
6. Good mornings for two repetitions

Today, with the heaviest weight you have used, do five sets.

High-repetition back squats

Today, try to get one set of 50 with the workout weight at the end of a heavy workout.

If you are 135 pounds or less, these are the weights you will use—

45 (the empty bar) x 10

45 (the empty bar) x 10

95 x 5

115 x 3

135 x 10

115 to fifty

If you are 135 to 185 pounds, these are the weights you will use—

45 x 5

135 x 5

135 x 3

185 x 10

135 x to fifty

If you are 185 to 205, you will use these weights—

     95 x 10

     135 x 5

     185 x 3

     205 x 10

     185 x to fifty

For everyone else, including guys who weigh a "lot" more, these are the weights—

     135 x 10

     185 x 2–3

     205 x 2–3

     225 x 10

     205 x to fifty

Cool-down

Take some time transitioning back to the real world. This is also a nice time to do anything you think you might need to do. I use this time for my corrective exercises for any injuries or issues that have appeared over the past season.

Program reminder

Tweak—Protein before and after this workout. Also, on that last set of the squat workout, do your best. If you can get all 50 reps, you are in rare air and well on your way to your lean body mass goals. Good luck!

General warm-up

1. Five minutes of gentle moving. Get the blood flowing.
2. Foam rolling (middle back, IT bands, hamstrings and hip flexors)
3. Static stretches for hip flexors, hamstrings, upper back and hot spots
4. Some easy swings, goblet squats and a few strides

Bench press

Please take a few minutes to warm up with appropriate light weights and prepare yourself for the heavier movements.

You have the option today of either going for an honest max single **OR** doing two sets of *2—3—5* with the weight you worked out with last time. The final set of five would indicate a major strength increase.

Max Bench: _____________________

2 x 2—3—5 with _____________________

Bat wings

Do five 10-second holds with your normal weight.

One-arm presses

Take a few easy warm-ups with lighter weights, then progress to your training weight. Try to stay with the heavier weights.

Begin with the weaker arm and do *2—3—5*.

Switch to the stronger arm and do *2—3—5*.

Repeat this for a total of two sets.

2—3—5 weight: _____________________, **two sets**

Bird dog

Practice the movement a few times. Do both sides and master the movement. Move your knees closer together over time.

Complex

A complex is a series of lifts back to back where you finish the reps of one lift before moving on to the next . The barbell only leaves your hands or touches the floor after all of the lifts are completed.

1. Row for two repetitions
2. Clean for two repetitions
3. Front squat for two repetitions
4. Military press for two repetitions
5. Back squat for two repetitions
6. Good mornings for two repetitions

This will be an easy day; use a "good" weight and just do three sets.

High-repetition back squats

Today, our goal is 50 reps with near bodyweight. Be sure to have good spotters.

If you are 135 pounds or less, these are the weights you will use—

45 (the empty bar) x 10

95 x 3

115 x 3

135 x to fifty

If you are 135 pounds to 185 pounds, these are the weights you will use—

45 x 5

135 x 5

135 x 3

185 x to fifty

If you are 185 to 205, you will use these weights—

95 x 10

135 x 5

185 x 3

205 x to fifty

For everyone else, including guys who weigh a "lot" more, these are the weights—

135 x 10

185 x 2–3

205 x 2–3

225 x to fifty

Cool-down

Take some time transitioning back to the real world. This is also a nice time to do any-thing you think you might need to do. I use this time for my corrective exercises for any injuries or issues that have appeared over the past season.

Congratulations. This is your final workout of the program.

If I ever recommended a workout that cut fat and built muscle at the same time, I'm not sure I'd believe myself. After all the late-night television hucksters, I'm not sure what to believe anymore.

But then, a student came up to me during the transition after our workout and asked, "Coach, can I get a copy of all the complexes for my dad? The rest of the guys in the fire department want to do them, too."

"Well, sure," I said. "Why?"

"Coach, everybody's getting huge."

So, without buying a plastic gizmo or a DVD of me in a tank top sweating to bad music, let's discuss complexes.

It all started when…

After eight years in a Catholic elementary school, I moved to a public junior high school and discovered how sheltered my life had been. Southwood Junior High in South San Francisco was a far cry from the quiet confines of my parish school with the good Irish nuns.

One thing we did have at Southwood was a fabulously simple weight training program.

Our Southwood workout, as I discussed in detail in and thread in my Q&A forum at *davedraper.com* (link below), was very straightforward.

Power clean x 8–6-4

Military press x 8–6-4

Front squat x 8–6-4

Bench press x 8–6-4

Here's the link to more detail:

http://www.davedraper.com/url/southwood.php

On one particular day due to a short class period for an assembly, our instructor, Mr. Freeman, simplified things even more. We just had to do power cleans, military presses and front squats for eight reps followed by a short rest as our partners did the three exercises. Then we'd do them for six reps before finishing with four.

Without the bench press, this workout sounded easy. He added one little thing, though: We couldn't put the bar down once we started the three lifts.

It's that back-to-back brutality that adds up, my friends. I choked on those last reps of the front squat trying to figure out where I left my lungs.

That was my first complex.

Going back in time

The roots of complexes are fairly deep, and reflect the peripheral heart action (PHA) workouts pioneered in the 1960s by Mr. America Bob Gajda, who also assisted the legendary Sergio Oliva. You can find more about it in John McCallum's great book, *Keys to Progress*.

Here's an example of one sequence from a PHA workout.

Front squat x 12

Cuddle sit-ups x 25

Curls x 10

Seated twists x 25

Wrestler's bridge x 10

Rest and repeat the sequence four total times. You'd then do up to three or four other sequences during this workout. It had advantages, as it seemed to burn a lot of fat and covered every body part imaginable.

There's an obvious problem with PHA. You have to have a lot of equipment; it's nice to be able to move from dumbbell to barbell to chin-up bar without having to wait or find the stuff you just left a minute ago. Those who train in college gyms or public establishments know that equipment will literally walk away to another corner as you move from exercise to exercise.

For many of us who trained in the 1970s, the Universal Gym was the answer to this problem. I had football workouts that were simply this—

Bench press

Lat pull-down

Leg press

Hyperextension

Leg extension and leg curl

Neck harness

Wrist roller

Shoulder press

Incline sit-up

After 30 seconds at each station, the coach would blow the whistle. We'd move over to the next position and continue training. This workout could accommodate a lot of athletes and, for what it was, this was a good workout.

The Nautilus machine workouts were also believed to improve cardiovascular condition by moving quickly from station to station. It allowed the gym owners to shuttle clients out of the gym quickly, too.

If you want to find out anything and everything under the sun about weightlifting, pop open your copy of John Jesse's *Wrestling Physical Conditioning Encyclopedia.* In its pages you'll find every variation, trick and special equipment ever conceived for strength training. The chapters on circuit training and endurance cover many of the basic principles of complexes.

In the past few years, Istvan "Steve" Javorek's work with complexes has been stolen and repackaged many times. I have to make a short nod to something he notes on his website—

> *"From what I've heard, from the far end of Siberia to Iceland to California, thousands of coaches are performing with their athletes Javorek's complex exercises, but some of them give credit to themselves. I really worked hard on developing these exercises and I like to share with everyone my 'little secrets.' Just give credit to the creator.*

> *"My original goal with the complex exercises was to find an efficient and aggressive method of performance enhancement that saves time and makes the program more enjoyable. If you choose to use these (in some form) with your athletes, be honest and call your new complex exercises 'Variation to Javorek's Complex Exercises.'"*

Javorek's complexes are brilliant and have all the keys to success for someone contemplating them.

Javorek's Barbell Complex #1

Barbell upright row x 6

Barbell high-pull snatch x 6

Barbell behind-the-head squat and push press x 6

Barbell behind-the-head good morning x 6

Barbell bent-over row x 6

You'll find the Javorek website at *istvanjavorek.com*; a few of the complexes are under the *sample exercises* link.

Another master of the complex is Alywn Cosgrove. On his recommendation, after the Velocity Diet, I began doing complexes and soon discovered not doing these on their own was one of the biggest oversights in my training career. I suggest you check your ego at the door before you begin complexes.

My definition of a complex is simple. A complex is a series of lifts back to back where you finish the reps of one lift before moving on to the next lift. The barbell only leaves your hands or touches the floor after all of the lifts are completed. Although you can do them with dumbbells or kettlebells, I argue to only use a barbell. Certainly there's great value in the other tools, but for getting athletes bigger, I like to use the heavier bar.

The key to organizing a complex is to make sure the bar passes over your head in some kind of logical manner. In other words, if you do rows first, followed by back squats, how did the bar get there? I try to have the bar pass backward over the head after a few lifts, but only pass forward again once.

When you try these, note that it'll save you some effort if you think about the exercise transitions before you get too heavy. For example, if you have a military press before a back squat, on the last military press rep, lower the weight to the back.

Take a minute to think these through before going for a max on these. In fact, it's probably best to use a broomstick first.

Your rest periods should be longer than what you might think. Like most of my workouts, these appear easy on paper.

The most difficult thing to consider is the rep range. For a fat-burning hit and a massive conditioning bang, try doing sets of eight.

Complex A for Eights

Row x 8

Clean x 8

Front squat x 8

Military press x 8

Back squat x 8

Good mornings x 8

Gently place the bar on the ground and rest!

I like sets of three for adding mass to my young athletes. The more time under the bar, the more the body adapts by getting bigger. Moreover, it seems to also be most helpful on the playing field. When you watch a sophomore boy handle Complex A with 155 for three segments of three reps each, you have to realize this is a very strong human being, even if he's just 15.

You can play with any rep variations you like, but I've found that eights and threes are the best. If you do five sets of eight, you probably won't be doing much more in this workout. Three sets of three make an excellent pre-lift warm-up, or, with heavier weights, can be used as a strength- and mass-building workout.

The sets seem to be almost geometric in the impact on the body. Err on the side of caution for the first few workouts before attempting more than three rounds.

An old variation, well, not terribly old, was used by greats such as Dave Draper as complexes for strength-building. Basically, in these we drop a rep each set and add weight. Now, be careful here, as the weights go up quickly.

Let's look at Complex C with this variation.

Complex C

Hang snatch

Overhead squat

Back squat

Good mornings

Row

Deadlift

Set 1: 8 reps with the bar, 45 pounds

Set 2: 7 reps with 65 pounds

Set 3: 6 reps with 85 pounds

Set 4: 5 reps with 105 pounds

Set 5: 4 reps with 125 pounds

Set 6: 3 reps with 145 pounds

Set 7: 2 reps with 165 pounds

Set 8: 1 rep with 185 pounds

There's an assumption here that you can snatch 185, then complete the workout. Again, on paper, this looks easy.

One other thing I like to do is print out each complex in size 68 Arial font so I can see the whole series on the ground in front of me. You'll find my complexes in full next, but if you want to print these out, go to *danjohn.net* and grab the *My Complexes* pdf near the top of the right sidebar. Print those out and place the sheet of the complex you're using about three feet in front of the barbell to help keep your mind on the exercise at hand. Use the sheet to remind you to move to the next exercise. With large groups, I have the sheets in plastic protectors, and reuse them for weeks at a time.

The Select Six

Now it's time I offer you my six favorite complexes. Note that each has six lifts—most of the exercises will be at least somewhat familiar to everyone. If you don't know how to do a lift, don't do it.

Complex A

Row

Clean

Front squat

Military press

Back squat

Good mornings

Complex B

Deadlift

Clean-grip high pull

Clean-grip snatch

Back squat

Good mornings

Row

Complex C

Hang snatch

Overhead squat

Back squat

Good mornings

Row

Deadlift

Complex D

Upright row

Clean-grip snatch

Back squat

Behind the neck press

Good mornings

Row

Complex E

Power clean

Military press

Back squat

Good mornings

Behind the neck press

Front squat

Complex F

Overhead squat

Back squat

Good morning

Front squat

Rows

Deadlift

Complexes: Keep it Simple

I find that swimming through these three times a week eliminates boredom. If you only do them twice a week and play with the three rep schemes (eights, threes and 8–7–6–5–4–3–2–1), you have 18 workout ideas that will last nine weeks.

When I sell this on late-night TV, I'll be the guy with the ponytail and spandex.

I am concerned about my body. I have lots of injuries and aches and pains and…

Hush. I understand. One of two things: either don't do it, which is what I suggest, or find a CK-FMS specialist. CK-FMS comprises a numbered screening system used by RKCs based on the Functional Movement Screen created by Gray Cook. If you have all "twos" and no asymmetries, you should be good to go. If not, seriously, do you really want to add more bulk to this beat-up body of yours?

Why are you such a jerk?

I'm not. I have just been doing this a long time and I know some people shouldn't/couldn't/wouldn't finish/attempt/try a program like this. So the illusion of me as a jerk seems to be true.

Well, you sound like a jerk.

True. Let's look at the three basic "truths" of my life in strength coaching—

1. Do no harm.
2. Ask the goal, then focus on the answer to the question *What is the goal?*
3. Follow a path toward that goal that has succeeded in other cases.

If you want to put on lean mass and you—

- Know how to squat
- Live basically pain-free
- Can handle the discipline of a six-week program

… and this book can help! If you want some cuddles and love, get a puppy.

I can't squat. What should I do? Are you willing to learn? *No.* Don't do this program.

I can't squat. What should I do? Are you willing to learn? *Yes.* It is going to suck, but do the six-week squat "education" program with just dumbbells or kettlebells. Train the rest of the body too, but give yourself some time to learn the squatting movement. If you can, get someone to teach you the basics of the back squat or use the resources on the internet. You can find my free one-hour squat clinic on my site at *danjohn.net.* Or you can purchase my DVDs covering the movement, like the four-part series from my Utah clinic or *From the Ground Up.*

I want to start taking this combination of supplements I saw at the [Local Nutrition Store] to help me put on mass. Why don't you recommend them?

There are magic powders that work. Sugar-free psyllium husk powders provide fiber. Quality protein powders can work miracles. Some guys do well with creatine.

Fish oil…well, it is an oil but pay attention: This is my one-stop shop for all and any issues. Others argue that probiotics can work miracles. Fine, take all of the above. But, then what?

Does eating steer testicles really work for humans? Does the berry of some rain forest tree really outgun eggs and toast? You see, I don't know. I don't think so, but I could be wrong. Again. But for most people, the answer is to save your money until you can back squat bodyweight for 50. Then, assess the magic powder again.

Hey, can I change this for that? (The five billion times I will answer this question will drive me crazy.)

No. Seriously. Remember how you adapted that other program and it failed miserably? Stop adapting. Follow the directions and do it exactly as written. If you take this system seriously, you will be stronger with surprisingly low volume and will gain lean body mass. Try it. After six weeks, then you can switch this for that.

You have lots of complexes listed in your website, articles and even here. Should I use these others?

No. I love them, too—like my children. Wait six weeks and then lose your mind with all the variations and variety. For now…focus.

Can I start this program and then do something else and come back to it?

Why, sure. Lots of people have died for you to have the freedom to do anything you want. I'm not sure it will work, but usually I can't stop people.

Why don't you do this? Start the program, focus on it with laser-beam intensity and finish it. Just a thought.

It's the end of the program. Now what?

First, go back and read the part beginning with *Week Seven: Assess,* page 54.

Literally, a thousand people who successfully finish the program may do a thousand different things after Week Six. Personally, I would suggest that you take the time to assess and come up with some insights about your progress. I would also suggest a look at your weaknesses either in strength or by body part. This is a great time to work on those issues.

Years ago I went on an interesting six-week fat-loss program where I stayed on the Atkins Induction of less than 20 grams of carbs a day for most of the week, and then had a carb feast on Friday night and all day Saturday. Sunday morning I looked forward to just eating bacon and eggs again. That program leaned me down to 209, the lightest I had been since nearly dying in Egypt—long story there.

The training was focused on my weakness: my arms! The program—

- Twice a week, Tiffini and I did three to five sets of arm curls and triceps extensions.
- One day a week, I did some squats, usually Tabata front squats. See this article for details: http://www.davedraper.com/url/tabata.php, but don't do the thrusters. That part was a bad idea.
- One other day a week, I did some military presses.

Yes, it was that simple. Of course, it worked so well, I stopped doing it! I have also experimented with the 40-day program after a hypertrophy phase that Pavel and I call Easy Strength. For more information about this, please get a copy of the book we co-wrote called *Easy Strength*.

But for now, here are the basics. A few years ago, Pavel outlined a simple program for me. Be wary, this program is so simple you'll ignore its value.

1. For the next 40 workouts, do the exact same training program every day. For the record, I find most of my goals are reached by day 20 or 22, so you can also opt for a shorter period.

2. Pick five exercises. I suggest a squatting movement like the goblet squat or overhead squat as part of the warm-up, as you don't want to ignore the movement. But it might be fun to focus on other aspects of your body.

3. Focus on these five movements—

- A large posterior-chain movement—the deadlift is the right answer

- Upper-body push—bench press, incline bench press, military press

- Upper-body pull—pull-ups, rows, or, if you've ignored them like I have, heavy biceps curls

- A full-body explosive move—kettlebell swings or snatches

- And something as an anterior-chain move—an abdominal exercise. I think the ab wheel is king here, but you can also do some other movements best suited for lower reps.

4. Only do two sets of five reps per workout for the deadlift and push/pull exercises, and one set of 20 to 50 for the explosive move. Do a solid single set of five reps for the abs.

5. Never plan or worry about the weight or the load. Always stay within yourself and go heavy naturally.

6. Don't eat chalk, scream or pound on walls. Do each lift without any emotion or excitement and strive for perfect technique.

It usually takes between eight and ten weeks to finish. Strive for five sessions a week, but variation will emerge. It's fine. It's life.

Of course, this can be an excellent prelude to the bulking program, too, if you know how to squat.

Dan, I feel fat and bloated. Are there any food issues I may be missing?

Whether you go low carb or eat whatever, I think most people would agree that to lean out, you have to reconsider reaching for boxes of insta-carbs and glasses of sugar-laden carbonated drinks. Remember the candy bar commercial a few years ago with the exhausted skier? He found that Brand X Candy gave him that instant energy to get him back on the slopes. The bar had 453 calories...more than two cans of tuna, almost three of some brands!

Call me when you get hungry after two cans of tuna.

So, let's at least agree to avoid the Evil Axis of Foods—

    1. Soft drinks—some argue even sugar-free drinks cause an insulin surge

    2. Candy bars, candies, candy-coated, sugar-coated, sugar-filled...by God, grow up and eat food!

    3. Chips, cookies and all the cardboard carbs

Cardboard carbohydrates are the carbs that come in boxes. They are processed, packaged and purified to go right to your hips and butt.

Let's add one area that Brian Oldfield, one of history's finest shot putters, explained as "one of the keys to performance." Simply, it is to learn what foods cause you to have an allergic reaction, or at the least, bother you a bit. If you ask the Lung Association, which has a long history with battling allergies, the answer will be simple: Peanuts, fish, egg, milk, wheat and soy cause most food allergies. Indeed, in the early 1980s, a popular muscle mag published an article saying 90 percent of Americans are allergic to wheat or milk.

I told this to a "nutritionist," who said this information is stupid because we find wheat products in everything, even McDonald's shakes. My first thought was: What kind of nutritionist thinks wheat products are in steak? Does a steer digest? It turns out she was wrong, at least now—corn is in every product.

Dr. Elson Haas notes in an interview with *Mind and Muscle Power* that the least allergic foods are rice, pears, lamb, kale, salmon and other deep sea fish, like halibut and sole, trout, turkey, rabbit, sweet potatoes and honey.

He goes on to recommend cabbage, carrots, cauliflower, broccoli, apricots, beets, squashes, olives, olive oil, cranberries, herbal teas and tapioca.

There are a number of books that give some ideas about eliminating problem foods. Many of us know from person experience that this or that food causes long-term problems. Anyone who has had trouble with allergies understands the need to stay clear of the troublemakers.

This isn't a judgment on certain foods. Not long ago, *Men's Journal* published a list of foods for muscle building—**The Superfoods:** eggs, almonds, salmon , yogurt, beef, olive oil, water, coffee. The list looks like my diet! While eggs may be poison to one person, they may be another's ticket to athletic success. Take some time to study your reactions to certain foods, consult a doctor who specializes in allergies, and fine-tune your diet.

Pavel gave this advice over a decade ago: *First, lay off the carbs. Eat steak. Read Anna Karenina for how long the Russian Officer Corps has been doing this. Eat your own breakfast, share your dinner and give your supper to an enemy. Third, build muscle. Fourth, do some cardio, but cycle your load.*

I think you knew the answer, didn't you?

Dan, what about steroids? Don't they add lean body weight faster than anything?

There are some "issues" with steroids. Here in the United States, they are seriously il-legal. They are banned by every sports federation I am involved with as a coach and athlete. Some argue they are immoral. Most agree they have long-term concerns, es-pecially in the area of heart health, but any of us who have been around long enough know the rest of the story.

I will answer the question in just a moment, but when I first started writing, it was a rare week when I didn't get an angry email from a guy, a famous name from back in the day, ranting about my comments on steroids. These would range from *I never did them* to *You can't compete without them* to *What the hell do you know, you never trained with me.* Then, he died. Sadly, these kinds of rants from former users now in middle age are more common than you would think. Another famous name once told me he got back on steroids as a very beat-up elderly athlete to get his bench press back over a certain number.

None of that is the issue. Here is the issue: If you do steroids, then what? Seriously, then what? One guy famously told elite athletes at the place that has the name for the sport-ing event held every four years that "steroids are the answer to all questions."

If you go down the dark side, then what? If you need anabolics to break 160 pounds of bodyweight or get a bodyweight squat, I can only imagine what you will need to do to make it to 180! So, stay clean for all the right reasons, but also for this one: Not doing steroids will give you a chance to tweak minor things that might give you some insights into how YOU grow.

What happens if I miss a day of training? Do I do it the next day? Will this throw off the whole six weeks?

The best thing to do is to not worry and do the workout the next day, have the day of rest, skip the recharge day and train again and get back on track. Ideally, you would only do this once in the six weeks. Now, if you can't help but have to skip days here and there, add a seventh week and do something like this—

> **Monday: Refresh and Recharge**
> **Tuesday: Train as indicated**
> **Wednesday: Rest**
> **Thursday: Recharge**
> **Friday: Rest**
> **Saturday: Train as indicated**
> **Sunday: Rest**

Keep the tweaks as indicated and use the last week to simply repeat the tweaks of Week Six and workouts 13 and 14. But try to do the six weeks as indicated. My feedback comes from people who followed the six weeks as noted in the materials here.

What do I do if I don't make the required reps? Or, what if I can't handle the weight I used the week before?

Well, that can happen. One of the best bits of feedback I received was from someone who had his bench go up so fast he started to turn this into the Wonderful Bench Improvement Protocol. Instead of dropping back as indicated, he decided to keep doing doubles with his max double. Bad idea, to say the least!

So, first, remember the program is based on the three components in combination: the upper body strength work, the complexes and the high-rep squats. The squats are the key. If you are handling the load there but having to go lighter in the other two pillars, you are still on the right track.

Also, it happens. You have a great day perhaps with the complexes and put on a load and crush it. A few days later, as we say: not so much…

Always feel free to lighten the load. I would rather see the weight on the bar a little less and have you finish all six weeks. It's okay to adjust. I would also take that mental time after a day or so and think about why you had to lighten up. It might be something easily fixable (more sleep needed, for example) and you can adjust.

In Conclusion

There will be some who will simply flip through this book and toss it back on the shelf and think, "Yeah, I knew all that." There will be others who will find a dozen problems and issues and reasons this six weeks of fun has to be adapted to this and that, which always results in doing the same nonproductive training as before reading it.

But a few, including the brave souls who have been my lab rats for this book, will insist on picking the book back up, gathering the tools needed and plugging away. Here is the overriding lesson for those who have tried this program: It is NOT the six weeks! It is what you LEARN about yourself.

I get the email messages telling me, "I can't believe what a difference a morning protein shake has made in my day; it's the best part of the program." The next email in the queue will tell me it was the shake before bed! Others note that it was the complexes or those odd *2—3—5* workouts.

It's the principles that are important here. Most trainees go through a long career without ever facing the bar to do 50 bodyweight squats and, maybe after doing it, discover NOT doing it was a better plan! But the exposure to these movements and the focus on one goal for six weeks will carry over in one's training.

Where you go from here is part of the wonderful journey of lifelong fitness. I guarantee this: After finishing the whole six weeks, you will have more clarity about work, rest and preparation than any other method I know.

If you finished it, congratulations—let me know how I can be of further service.

If you are on the path to finishing, I may not be in the weightroom with you, but please know that I am cheering you on all the way.

Good luck and… Never Let Go.

Dan John

	Monday	Tuesday	Wednesday	Thursday	Friday	Saturday	Sunday
Week 1	Train **Day 1**	Rest	Recharge	Train **Day 2**	Rest	Recharge	Train **Day 3**
Week 2	Rest	Recharge	Train **Day 4**	Rest	Recharge	Train **Day 5**	Rest
Week 3	Recharge	Train **Day 6**	Rest	Recharge	Train **Day 7**	Rest	Recharge
Week 4	Train **Day 8**	Rest	Recharge	Train **Day 9**	Rest	Recharge	Train **Day 10**
Week 5	Rest	Recharge	Train **Day 11**	Rest	Recharge	Train **Day 12**	Rest
Week 6	Recharge	Train **Day 13**	Rest	Recharge	Train **Day 14**	Rest	Recharge
Week 7	**Assess the program**						

Week One

Monday: Training Day One

Tuesday: Rest

Wednesday: Recharge

Thursday: Training Day Two

Friday: Rest

Saturday: Recharge

Sunday: Training Day Three

Beginning weight, Monday ___________

Nutritional instructions:

> **Begin experimenting with three meals and multiple daily snacks—see page 51.**

WEEK ONE, MONDAY — TRAINING DAY ONE   DATE __________________________

General warm-up
- ☐ Five minutes of gentle moving—get the blood flowing
- ☐ Foam rolling (middle back, IT band, hamstrings and hip flexors)
- ☐ Static stretches for hip flexors, hamstrings, upper back and hot spots
- ☐ Some easy swings, goblet squats and a few strides

Bench Press: *Warm-ups then...*

	Weight used		**Weight used**
Easy weight, set of 5		*Add weight, set of 5*	
Add weight, set of 5		*Add weight, set of 5*	
Add weight, set of 5		*Add weight, set of 5*	
Final weight, set of 5			
Record this final weight __________			

Bat Wings: *Testing weights*

10-second holds	*Test 1:*	*Test 2:*	*Test 3:*
Record this final weight __________			

One-Arm Press: *Testing weights, starting with the weaker arm*

2-3 reps each arm	*Test 1:*	*Test 2:*	*Test 3:*
Record this final weight __________			

Bird Dog: *Practice the movement on both sides, moving your knees closer together over time.*
Complex: *Do three repetitions of each exercises. Add a little weight and repeat for a total of three rounds. Record the weight used in each round.*

Row | Clean | Front Squat | Military Press | Back Squat | Good Morning

Round 1:		*Round 2:*		*Round 3:*	

High-Rep Back Squats: *One set of 30 with 95 pounds—if you're lighter than 135, use an empty bar.*

Cool-down: *Record your personal cool-down plan of stretching or corrective exercises.*

____

____

Nutritional compliance (Y/N) _____ More protein _____ More fiber _____ More fish oil

WEEK ONE, TUESDAY — REST DATE ________________________

Shop, organize, prepare food

Nutritional compliance (Y/N) _______ More protein _______ More fiber _______ More fish oil

Other thoughts ____

____

____

WEEK ONE, WEDNESDAY — RECHARGE DATE ________________________

Your choice of 10-20 minutes of quality, low-intensity movement. Record your exercise choices and movement quality discoveries, and remember to note things to work on next *Recharge* day.

____

____

____

____

____

____

Nutritional compliance (Y/N) _______ More protein _______ More fiber _______ More fish oil

Other thoughts ____

____

____

WEEK ONE, THURSDAY — TRAINING DAY TWO   DATE _______________________

General warm-up
- ☐ Five minutes of gentle moving—get the blood flowing
- ☐ Foam rolling (middle back, IT band, hamstrings and hip flexors)
- ☐ Static stretches for hip flexors, hamstrings, upper back and hot spots
- ☐ Some easy swings, goblet squats and a few strides

Bench Press: *Warm-ups then… 2—3—5. With the weight from the last workout, do:*

	Weight used
Two reps, rest a little. Three reps, rest a little. Five reps, rest a little.	
Two reps, rest a little. Three reps, rest a little. Five reps, rest a little.	

Bat Wings: *Using the weight from Day One…*

10 five-second holds with:									

One-Arm Press: *Light warm-up, then, use the weight from Day One. Start on the weaker arm.*

	Weight used
Two reps, rest a little. Three reps, rest a little. Five reps, rest a little.	
Two reps, rest a little. Three reps, rest a little. Five reps, rest a little.	

Bird Dog: *Practice the movement on both sides, moving your knees closer together over time.*

Complex: *Do three repetitions of each exercises. Repeat for a total of five rounds. Add a little weight after the first three rounds. The final weight is your starting weight next workout.*

Row	Clean	Front Squat	Military Press	Back Squat	Good Morning
Round 1:	*Round 2:*	*Round 3:*	*Round 4:*	*Round 5:*	

High-Rep Back Squats: *See page 71 for weight instructions.*

2 sets of 30 reps — Record your weights used here: ___________ | ___________

Cool-down: *Record your personal cool-down plan of stretching or corrective exercises.*

____

____

Nutritional compliance (Y/N) ______ More protein ______ More fiber ______ More fish oil

WEEK ONE, FRIDAY — REST   DATE _______________________________

Shop, organize, prepare food

Nutritional compliance (Y/N) _______ More protein _______ More fiber _______ More fish oil

Other thoughts ____

____

____

WEEK ONE, SATURDAY — RECHARGE   DATE _______________________________

Your choice of 10-20 minutes of quality, low-intensity movement. Record your exercise choices and movement quality discoveries, and remember to note things to work on next *Recharge* **day.**

____

____

____

____

____

Nutritional compliance (Y/N) _______ More protein _______ More fiber _______ More fish oil

Other thoughts ____

____

WEEK ONE, SUNDAY — TRAINING DAY THREE   DATE ______________________

General warm-up

- ☐ Five minutes of gentle moving—get the blood flowing
- ☐ Foam rolling (middle back, IT band, hamstrings and hip flexors)
- ☐ Static stretches for hip flexors, hamstrings, upper back and hot spots
- ☐ Some easy swings, goblet squats and a few strides

Bench Press: *Warm-ups then… 2—3—5. With the weight from the last workout, do:*

	Weight used
Two reps, rest a little. Three reps, rest a little. Five reps, rest a little.	
Two reps, rest a little. Three reps, rest a little. Five reps, rest a little.	
Two reps, rest a little. Three reps, rest a little. Five reps, rest a little.	
If all reps completed, next workout move up to:	

Bat Wings: *Using the weight from Day One…*

10 five-second holds with:									

One-Arm Press: *Light warm-up, then, use the weight from Day One. Start on the weaker arm.*

	Weight used
Two reps, rest a little. Three reps, rest a little. Five reps, rest a little.	
Two reps, rest a little. Three reps, rest a little. Five reps, rest a little.	
Two reps, rest a little. Three reps, rest a little. Five reps, rest a little.	
If all reps completed, next workout move up to:	

Bird Dog: *Practice the movement on both sides, moving your knees closer together over time.*

Complex: *Do five repetitions of each exercises. Repeat for a total of two rounds.*

Row | Clean | Front Squat | Military Press | Back Squat | Good Morning

Round 1:	*Round 2:*

High-Rep Back Squats: *See page 73 for weight instructions.*

2 sets of 30 reps — Record your weights used here:_____________ | _____________

Cool-down: *Record your personal cool-down plan of stretching or corrective exercises.*

____

____

Nutritional compliance (Y/N) ______ More protein ______ More fiber ______ More fish oil

Week Two

Monday: Rest

Tuesday: Recharge

Wednesday: Training Day Four

Thursday: Rest

Friday: Recharge

Saturday: Training Day Five

Sunday: Rest

Beginning weight, Monday ___________

Nutritional instructions:

Drink a protein shake before going to bed—see page 51.

Program Tweaks:

There are only two workouts this week, but a lot of additional protein. This is an important week to track moods and size gains.

WEEK TWO, MONDAY — REST   DATE _______________________________

Shop, organize, prepare food

Nutritional compliance (Y/N) ______ More protein ______ More fiber ______ More fish oil

Other thoughts ____

____

____

WEEK TWO, TUESDAY — RECHARGE   **DATE** _______________________________

Your choice of 10-20 minutes of quality, low-intensity movement. Record your exercise choices and movement quality discoveries, and remember to note things to work on next *Recharge* day.

____

____

____

____

____

Nutritional compliance (Y/N) ______ More protein ______ More fiber ______ More fish oil

Other thoughts ____

____

WEEK TWO, WEDNESDAY — TRAINING DAY FOUR   DATE __________________

General warm-up

- ☐ Five minutes of gentle moving—get the blood flowing
- ☐ Foam rolling (middle back, IT band, hamstrings and hip flexors)
- ☐ Static stretches for hip flexors, hamstrings, upper back and hot spots
- ☐ Some easy swings, goblet squats and a few strides

Bench Press: *Warm-ups then… 2—3—5. Then, with the old weight from last Sunday, do as many as up to 10:*

	Weight used
Two reps, rest a little. Three reps, rest a little. Five reps, rest a little.	
Two reps, rest a little. Three reps, rest a little. Five reps, rest a little.	
With the old weight from last Sunday, do as many reps as 10	

Bat Wings: *Using the weight from Day One…*

Five 10-second holds with:				

One-Arm Press: *Light warm-up, then, use the weight from Day One. Start on the weaker arm.*

	Weight used
Two reps, rest a little. Three reps, rest a little. Five reps, rest a little.	
Two reps, rest a little. Three reps, rest a little. Five reps, rest a little.	

Bird Dog: *Practice the movement on both sides, moving your knees closer together over time.*

Complex: *Finish all reps of each exercise before moving on. Repeat for a total of three rounds. Use the weight you handled Sunday.*

Row	**Clean**	**Front Squat**	**Military Press**	**Back Squat**	**Good Morning**
Round 1:		*Round 2:*		*Round 3:*	

High-Rep Back Squats: *See page 75 for weight instructions.*

3 sets of 30 reps — Record your weights used here:__________ | __________ | __________

Cool-down: *Record your personal cool-down plan of stretching or corrective exercises.*

____

____

Nutritional compliance (Y/N) _____ More protein _____ More fiber _____ More fish oil

WEEK TWO, THURSDAY — REST   DATE _______________________________

Shop, organize, prepare food

Nutritional compliance (Y/N) _______ More protein _______ More fiber _______ More fish oil

Other thoughts ____

____

____

WEEK TWO, FRIDAY — RECHARGE   DATE _______________________________

Your choice of 10-20 minutes of quality, low-intensity movement. Record your exercise choices and movement quality discoveries, and remember to note things to work on next *Recharge* day.

____

____

____

____

____

Nutritional compliance (Y/N) _______ More protein _______ More fiber _______ More fish oil

Other thoughts ____

____

WEEK TWO, SATURDAY — TRAINING DAY FIVE   DATE _______________________

General warm-up

- ☐ Five minutes of gentle moving—get the blood flowing
- ☐ Foam rolling (middle back, IT band, hamstrings and hip flexors)
- ☐ Static stretches for hip flexors, hamstrings, upper back and hot spots
- ☐ Some easy swings, goblet squats and a few strides

Bench Press: *Warm-ups then… 2—3—5. With the new goal weight used last workout, do:*

	Weight used
Two reps, rest a little. Three reps, rest a little. Five reps, rest a little.	
Two reps, rest a little. Three reps, rest a little. Five reps, rest a little.	
Two reps, rest a little. Three reps, rest a little. Five reps, rest a little.	

Bat Wings: *Using a heavier weight this time… Really try to squeeze the shoulder blades together.*

Five 5-second holds with:					

One-Arm Press: *Light warm-up, then, use the weight from Day One. Start on the weaker arm.*

	Weight used
Two reps, rest a little. Three reps, rest a little. Five reps, rest a little.	
Two reps, rest a little. Three reps, rest a little. Five reps, rest a little.	
Two reps, rest a little. Three reps, rest a little. Five reps, rest a little.	

Bird Dog: *Practice the movement on both sides, moving your knees closer together over time.*

Complex: *Do five repetitions of each exercise. Repeat for a total of three rounds.*
Use the weight you handled last time.

Row	Clean	Front Squat	Military Press	Back Squat	Good Morning

Round 1:	*Round 2:*	*Round 3:*

High-Rep Back Squats: *See page 77-78 for weight AND set/rep instructions.*

Record your weights and reps here:___________ | ___________ | ___________ | ___________

Cool-down: *Record your personal cool-down plan of stretching or corrective exercises.*

____

____

Nutritional compliance (Y/N) _____ More protein _____ More fiber _____ More fish oil

WEEK TWO, SUNDAY — REST   DATE ______________________________

Shop, organize, prepare food

Nutritional compliance (Y/N) _______ More protein _______ More fiber _______ More fish oil

Other thoughts ____

____

____

As we end week two, make note of what seems to be working or not working for you.

____

____

____

____

____

____

____

____

____

Week Three

Monday: Recharge

Tuesday: Training Day Six

Wednesday: Rest

Thursday: Recharge

Friday: Training Day Seven

Saturday: Rest

Sunday: Recharge

Beginning weight, Monday ___________

Nutritional instructions:

Add an additional scoop of protein just prior to training—see page 52.

Program Tweaks:

There are only two workouts this week, but a lot of additional protein. This, too, is an important week to track moods and size gains.

Your choice of 10-20 minutes of quality, low-intensity movement. Record your exercise choices and movement quality discoveries, and remember to note things to work on next *Recharge* **day.**

____

____

____

____

Anything you tried and need to remember from yesterday's notes?

____

____

____

____

Nutritional compliance (Y/N) ______ More protein ______ More fiber ______ More fish oil

Other thoughts ____

____

WEEK THREE, TUESDAY — TRAINING DAY SIX   DATE __________________

General warm-up

- ☐ Five minutes of gentle moving—get the blood flowing
- ☐ Foam rolling (middle back, IT band, hamstrings and hip flexors)
- ☐ Static stretches for hip flexors, hamstrings, upper back and hot spots
- ☐ Some easy swings, goblet squats and a few strides

Bench Press: *Warm-ups then… 2—3—5—10. With the new goal weight used last workout, do:*

	Weight used
Two reps, rest a little. Three reps, rest a little. Five reps, rest a little. Up to 10.	
Two reps, rest a little. Three reps, rest a little. Five reps, rest a little.	
Two reps, rest a little. Three reps, rest a little. Five reps, rest a little.	

Bat Wings: *Using a heavier weight this time… Really try to squeeze the shoulder blades together.*

Five 5-second holds with:					

One-Arm Press: *Light warm-up, then, try to use a heavier weight. Start on the weaker arm.*

	Weight used
Two reps, rest a little. Three reps, rest a little. Five reps, rest a little.	
Two reps, rest a little. Three reps, rest a little. Five reps, rest a little.	
Two reps, rest a little. Three reps, rest a little. Five reps, rest a little.	

Bird Dog: *Practice the movement on both sides, moving your knees closer together over time.*

Complex: *Do five repetitions of each exercise. Repeat for a total of five rounds. Use the weight you handled last time if possible, but going lighter on the first and last set is also okay.*

Row	Clean	Front Squat	Military Press	Back Squat	Good Morning
Round 1:		*Round 2:*	*Round 3:*	*Round 4:*	*Round 5:*

High-Rep Back Squats *to Fifty*: *See page 80-81 for weight AND set/rep instructions.*

Record your weights and reps here:___________ | __________ | __________ | ________

Cool-down: *Record your personal cool-down plan of stretching or corrective exercises.*

____

____

Nutritional compliance (Y/N) ______ More protein ______ More fiber ______ More fish oil

WEEK THREE, WEDNESDAY — REST   DATE _______________________________

Shop, organize, prepare food

Nutritional compliance (Y/N) ______ More protein ______ More fiber ______ More fish oil

Other thoughts ____

____

____

WEEK THREE, THURSDAY — RECHARGE   DATE _______________________________

Your choice of 10-20 minutes of quality, low-intensity movement. Record your exercise choices and movement quality discoveries, and remember to note things to work on next *Recharge* **day.**

____

____

____

____

____

Nutritional compliance (Y/N) ______ More protein ______ More fiber ______ More fish oil

Other thoughts ____

____

WEEK THREE, FRIDAY — TRAINING DAY SEVEN   DATE ______________________

General warm-up

- ☐ Five minutes of gentle moving—get the blood flowing
- ☐ Foam rolling (middle back, IT band, hamstrings and hip flexors)
- ☐ Static stretches for hip flexors, hamstrings, upper back and hot spots
- ☐ Some easy swings, goblet squats and a few strides

Bench Press: *Warm-ups then… It's Max Doubles. We're looking for two clean, heavy reps.*

	Weight used
Today's Max Double	

Bat Wings: *Using the same weight as last workout… Squeeze the shoulder blades together.*

Five 10-second holds with:				

One-Arm Press: *Light warm-up, then use the same weight as last time. Start on the weaker arm.*

	Weight used
Two reps, rest a little. Three reps, rest a little. Five reps, rest a little.	
Two reps, rest a little. Three reps, rest a little. Five reps, rest a little.	

Bird Dog: *Practice the movement on both sides, moving your knees closer together over time.*

Complex: *Do five repetitions of each exercise. Repeat for a total of three rounds. Move the weight up each set.*

Row | Clean | Front Squat | Military Press | Back Squat | Good Morning

Round 1:	*Round 2:*	*Round 3:*

High-Rep Back Squats: *See page 83-84 for weight AND set/rep instructions.*

Record your weights and reps here: __________ | __________ | __________ | __________

__________ | __________ | __________ | __________

Cool-down: *Record your personal cool-down plan of stretching or corrective exercises.*

____

____

Nutritional compliance (Y/N) _____ More protein _____ More fiber _____ More fish oil

WEEK THREE, SATURDAY — REST   DATE _______________________________

Shop, organize, prepare food

Nutritional compliance (Y/N) _______ More protein _______ More fiber _______ More fish oil

Other thoughts ____

____

____

WEEK THREE, SUNDAY — RECHARGE   DATE _______________________________

Your choice of 10-20 minutes of quality, low-intensity movement. Record your exercise choices and movement quality discoveries, and remember to note things to work on next *Recharge* day.

____

____

____

____

____

Nutritional compliance (Y/N) _______ More protein _______ More fiber _______ More fish oil

Other thoughts ____

____

Week Four

Monday: Training Day Eight

Tuesday: Rest

Wednesday: Recharge

Thursday: Training Day Nine

Friday: Rest

Saturday: Recharge

Sunday: Training Day Ten

Beginning weight, Monday _____________

Nutritional instructions:

 Add five grams of creatine daily—see page 53.

WEEK FOUR, MONDAY — TRAINING DAY EIGHT   DATE ________________

General warm-up

- ☐ Five minutes of gentle moving—get the blood flowing
- ☐ Foam rolling (middle back, IT band, hamstrings and hip flexors)
- ☐ Static stretches for hip flexors, hamstrings, upper back and hot spots
- ☐ Some easy swings, goblet squats and a few strides

Bench Press: *Warm-ups then… 5 sets of 2 reps with 20 pounds less than Friday's Max Double.*

Weight used for 5 sets of 2 reps				

Bat Wings: *Using the same weight… or you can experiment with a heavier weight.*

Five 10-second holds with:				

One-Arm Press: *Light warm-up, then use the same weight as last time. Start on the weaker arm.*

	Weight used
Two reps, rest a little. Three reps, rest a little. Five reps, rest a little.	
Two reps, rest a little. Three reps, rest a little. Five reps, rest a little.	

Bird Dog: *Practice the movement on both sides, moving your knees closer together over time.*

Complex: *Do two repetitions of each exercise. Repeat for a total of five rounds. Move the weight up each set.*

Row	**Clean**	**Front Squat**	**Military Press**	**Back Squat**	**Good Morning**
Round 1:	*Round 2:*	*Round 3:*	*Round 4:*	*Round 5:*	

High-Rep Back Squats *to Fifty*: *See page 86-87 for weight AND set/rep instructions.*

Record your weights and reps here: _________ | _________ | _________ | _________

_________ | _________ | _________ | _________

Cool-down: *Record your personal cool-down plan of stretching or corrective exercises.*

____

____

Nutritional compliance (Y/N) ______ More protein ______ More fiber ______ More fish oil

WEEK FOUR, TUESDAY — REST DATE __________________________

Shop, organize, prepare food

Nutritional compliance (Y/N) _____ More protein _____ More fiber _____ More fish oil

Other thoughts ____

____

____

WEEK FOUR, WEDNESDAY — RECHARGE DATE _________________________

Your choice of 10-20 minutes of quality, low-intensity movement. Record your exercise choices and movement quality discoveries, and remember to note things to work on next *Recharge* **day.**

____

____

____

____

____

Nutritional compliance (Y/N) _____ More protein _____ More fiber _____ More fish oil

Other thoughts ____

____

____

WEEK FOUR, THURSDAY — TRAINING DAY NINE   DATE_______________________

General warm-up
- ☐ Five minutes of gentle moving—get the blood flowing
- ☐ Foam rolling (middle back, IT band, hamstrings and hip flexors)
- ☐ Static stretches for hip flexors, hamstrings, upper back and hot spots
- ☐ Some easy swings, goblet squats and a few strides

Bench Press: *Warm-ups then… 5 sets of 3 reps with 20 pounds less than Friday's Max Double.*

Weight used for 5 sets of 3 reps				

Bat Wings: *Using the same weight… or you can experiment with a heavier weight.*

Five 10-second holds with:				

One-Arm Press: *Light warm-up, then use the same weight as last time. Start on the weaker arm.*

	Weight used
Two reps, rest a little. Three reps, rest a little. Five reps, rest a little.	
Two reps, rest a little. Three reps, rest a little. Five reps, rest a little.	
Two reps, rest a little. Three reps, rest a little. Five reps, rest a little.	

Bird Dog: *Practice the movement on both sides, moving your knees closer together over time.*

Complex: *Do two repetitions of each exercise. Repeat for a total of three rounds.*
Start with the weight you ended with on Monday, and move the weight up each set.

Row	Clean	Front Squat	Military Press	Back Squat	Good Morning

Round 1:	Round 2:	Round 3:

High-Rep Back Squats: *See page 89-90 for weight AND set/rep instructions.*

Record your weights and reps here: _________ | _________ | _________ | _________

_________ | _________ | _________ | _________

Cool-down: *Record your personal cool-down plan of stretching or corrective exercises.*

____

____

Nutritional compliance (Y/N) ______ More protein ______ More fiber ______ More fish oil

WEEK FOUR, FRIDAY — REST   DATE ________________________

Shop, organize, prepare food

Nutritional compliance (Y/N) ______ More protein ______ More fiber ______ More fish oil

Other thoughts ____

____

____

WEEK FOUR, SATURDAY — RECHARGE   DATE ________________________

Your choice of 10-20 minutes of quality, low-intensity movement. Record your exercise choices and movement quality discoveries, and remember to note things to work on next *Recharge* day.

____

____

____

____

Nutritional compliance (Y/N) ______ More protein ______ More fiber ______ More fish oil

Other thoughts ____

____

WEEK FOUR, SUNDAY — TRAINING DAY TEN   DATE _______________________

General warm-up

- ☐ Five minutes of gentle moving—get the blood flowing
- ☐ Foam rolling (middle back, IT band, hamstrings and hip flexors)
- ☐ Static stretches for hip flexors, hamstrings, upper back and hot spots
- ☐ Some easy swings, goblet squats and a few strides

Bench Press: *Warm-ups then… using the weight from the last two workout, two sets of 2—3—5.*

	Weight used
Two reps, rest a little. Three reps, rest a little. Five reps, rest a little.	
Two reps, rest a little. Three reps, rest a little. Five reps, rest a little.	

Bat Wings: *Using a heavier weight….*

Five 10-second holds with:					

One-Arm Press: *Light warm-up, then use the same weight as last time. Start on the weaker arm.*

	Weight used
Two reps, rest a little. Three reps, rest a little. Five reps, rest a little.	
Two reps, rest a little. Three reps, rest a little. Five reps, rest a little.	

Bird Dog: *Practice the movement on both sides, moving your knees closer together over time.*

Complex: *Do two repetitions of each exercise. Repeat for a total of five rounds.*
Use the heaviest weight from Thursday.

Row	Clean	Front Squat	Military Press	Back Squat	Good Morning
Round 1:	*Round 2:*	*Round 3:*	*Round 4:*	*Round 5:*	

High-Rep Back Squats *to Fifty:* *See page 92-93 for weight AND set/rep instructions.*

Record your weights and reps here: _________ | _________ | _________ | _________

Cool-down: *Record your personal cool-down plan of stretching or corrective exercises.*

____

____

Nutritional compliance (Y/N) ______ More protein ______ More fiber ______ More fish oil

Week Five

Monday: Rest

Tuesday: Recharge

Wednesday: Training Day Eleven

Thursday: Rest

Friday: Recharge

Saturday: Training Day Twelve

Sunday: Rest

Beginning weight, Monday ____________

Nutritional instructions:

Add a two-scoop protein shake upon rising daily—see page 53.

Program Tweaks:
If you are following the tweaks exactly, today…beyond meals and snacks…you will have five scoops of protein and some creatine. Let's make some progress!

WEEK FIVE, MONDAY — REST   DATE _______________________________

Shop, organize, prepare food

Nutritional compliance (Y/N) _______ More protein _______ More fiber _______ More fish oil

Other thoughts ____

____

____

WEEK FIVE, TUESDAY — RECHARGE   DATE _______________________________

Your choice of 10-20 minutes of quality, low-intensity movement. Record your exercise choices and movement quality discoveries, and remember to note things to work on next *Recharge* day.

____

____

____

____

____

____

Nutritional compliance (Y/N) _______ More protein _______ More fiber _______ More fish oil

Other thoughts ____

____

____

General warm-up
- ☐ Five minutes of gentle moving—get the blood flowing
- ☐ Foam rolling (middle back, IT band, hamstrings and hip flexors)
- ☐ Static stretches for hip flexors, hamstrings, upper back and hot spots
- ☐ Some easy swings, goblet squats and a few strides

Bench Press: *Warm-ups then… It's Max Doubles. We're looking for two clean, heavy reps.*

	Weight used
Today's Max Double	

Bat Wings: *Using a heavier weight….*

Five 10-second holds with:					

One-Arm Press: *Light warm-up, then use the same weight as last time. Start on the weaker arm.*

	Weight used
Two reps, rest a little. Three reps, rest a little. Five reps, rest a little.	
Two reps, rest a little. Three reps, rest a little. Five reps, rest a little.	

Bird Dog: *Practice the movement on both sides, moving your knees closer together over time.*

Complex: *Do five repetitions of each exercise. Repeat for a total of three rounds. Start with a lighter weight on the first sent and try to match last workout's weight on the final sets.*

Row	Clean	Front Squat	Military Press	Back Squat	Good Morning
Round 1:		*Round 2:*		*Round 3:*	

High-Rep Back Squats *to Fifty:* **See page 95-96 for weight AND set/rep instructions.**

Record your weights and reps here: ___________ | ___________ | ___________ | ___________

Cool-down: *Record your personal cool-down plan of stretching or corrective exercises.*

____

____

Nutritional compliance (Y/N) ______ More protein ______ More fiber ______ More fish oil

WEEK FIVE, THURSDAY — REST   DATE ______________________________

Shop, organize, prepare food

Nutritional compliance (Y/N) _______ More protein _______ More fiber _______ More fish oil

Other thoughts ____

____

____

WEEK FIVE, FRIDAY — RECHARGE   DATE ______________________________

Your choice of 10-20 minutes of quality, low-intensity movement. Record your exercise choices and movement quality discoveries, and remember to note things to work on next *Recharge* day.

____

____

____

____

____

Nutritional compliance (Y/N) _______ More protein _______ More fiber _______ More fish oil

Other thoughts ____

____

WEEK FIVE, SATURDAY — TRAINING DAY TWELVE   DATE _______________________

General warm-up
- ☐ Five minutes of gentle moving—get the blood flowing
- ☐ Foam rolling (middle back, IT band, hamstrings and hip flexors)
- ☐ Static stretches for hip flexors, hamstrings, upper back and hot spots
- ☐ Some easy swings, goblet squats and a few strides

Bench Press: *Warm-ups then… 5 sets of 2 reps with 20 pounds less than Wednesday's Max Double.*

Weight used for 5 sets of 2 reps				

Bat Wings: *Using a heavier weight….*

Five 5-10-second holds with:				

One-Arm Press: *Light warm-up, then use the same weight as last time. Start on the weaker arm.*

	Weight used
Two reps, rest a little. Three reps, rest a little. Five reps, rest a little.	
Two reps, rest a little. Three reps, rest a little. Five reps, rest a little.	
Two reps, rest a little. Three reps, rest a little. Five reps, rest a little.	

Bird Dog: *Practice the movement on both sides, moving your knees closer together over time.*

Complex: *Do **three** repetitions of each exercise. Repeat for a total of three rounds.
Use the heaviest weight you used Wednesday.*

Row	Clean	Front Squat	Military Press	Back Squat	Good Morning
Round 1:			*Round 2:*		*Round 3:*

High-Rep Back Squats *to Fifty*: *See page 98 -99 for weight AND set/rep instructions.*

Record your weights and reps here: ___________ | ___________ | ___________ | ___________

Cool-down: *Record your personal cool-down plan of stretching or corrective exercises.*

____

____

Nutritional compliance (Y/N) ______ More protein ______ More fiber ______ More fish oil

Shop, organize, prepare food

Nutritional compliance (Y/N) _______ More protein _______ More fiber _______ More fish oil

Other thoughts ____

____

____

As we end week five with one week to go, take some time to refocus in order to end fully engaged. Make note of anything you think of that's been holding you back, or that you've been neglecting so you can fix them in the upcoming final week push.

____

____

____

____

____

____

____

____

Week Six

Monday: Recharge

Tuesday: Training Day Thirteen

Wednesday: Rest

Thursday: Recharge

Friday: Training Day Fourteen

Saturday: Rest

Sunday: Recharge

Beginning weight, Monday _____________

Nutritional instructions:

Add a one-scoop protein drink after finishing your workouts—see page 54.

Your choice of 10-20 minutes of quality, low-intensity movement. Record your exercise choices and movement quality discoveries, and remember to note things to work on next *Recharge* day.

____

____

____

____

Anything you need to remember from yesterday's notes to help make this week a success?

____

____

____

____

Nutritional compliance (Y/N) ______ More protein ______ More fiber ______ More fish oil

Other thoughts ____

____

____

WEEK SIX, TUESDAY — TRAINING DAY THIRTEEN   DATE ______________________

General warm-up

- ☐ Five minutes of gentle moving—get the blood flowing
- ☐ Foam rolling (middle back, IT band, hamstrings and hip flexors)
- ☐ Static stretches for hip flexors, hamstrings, upper back and hot spots
- ☐ Some easy swings, goblet squats and a few strides

Bench Press: *Warm-ups then… 5 sets of 3 reps with the same weight as last Saturday.*

Weight used for 5 sets of 3 reps				

Bat Wings: *Using your normal weight….*

Five 10-second holds with:				

One-Arm Press: *Light warm-up, then try to move to a heavier weight. Start on the weaker arm.*

	Weight used
Two reps, rest a little. Three reps, rest a little. Five reps, rest a little.	
Two reps, rest a little. Three reps, rest a little. Five reps, rest a little.	
Two reps, rest a little. Three reps, rest a little. Five reps, rest a little.	

Bird Dog: *Practice the movement on both sides, moving your knees closer together over time.*

Complex: *Do **two** repetitions of each exercise. Repeat for a total of five rounds.*
Use the heaviest weight you've used.

Row	Clean	Front Squat	Military Press	Back Squat	Good Morning
Round 1:	*Round 2:*	*Round 3:*	*Round 4:*	*Round 5:*	

High-Rep Back Squats *to Fifty*: *See page 101-102 for weight AND set/rep instructions.*

Record your weights and reps here: __________ | __________ | __________ | __________

__________ | __________ | __________ | __________

Cool-down: *Record your personal cool-down plan of stretching or corrective exercises.*

____

____

Nutritional compliance (Y/N) ______ More protein ______ More fiber ______ More fish oil

WEEK SIX, WEDNESDAY — REST   DATE ______________________________

Shop, organize, prepare food

Nutritional compliance (Y/N) ______ More protein ______ More fiber ______ More fish oil

Other thoughts ____

____

____

WEEK SIX, THURSDAY — RECHARGE   DATE ______________________

Your choice of 10-20 minutes of quality, low-intensity movement. Record your exercise choices and movement quality discoveries, and remember to note things to work on next *Recharge* day.

____

____

____

____

____

Nutritional compliance (Y/N) ______ More protein ______ More fiber ______ More fish oil

Other thoughts ____

____

____

WEEK SIX, FRIDAY — TRAINING DAY FOURTEEN   DATE ________________

General warm-up

- ☐ Five minutes of gentle moving—get the blood flowing
- ☐ Foam rolling (middle back, IT band, hamstrings and hip flexors)
- ☐ Static stretches for hip flexors, hamstrings, upper back and hot spots
- ☐ Some easy swings, goblet squats and a few strides

Bench Press: *Warm-ups then… see page 103 for your bench press choice.*

Max Bench:________________   *or*

	Weight used
Two reps, rest a little. Three reps, rest a little. Five reps, rest a little. Up to 10.	
Two reps, rest a little. Three reps, rest a little. Five reps, rest a little.	

Bat Wings: *Using your normal weight….*

Five 10-second holds with:				

One-Arm Press: *Light warm-up, then try to stay with a heavier weight. Start on the weaker arm.*

	Weight used
Two reps, rest a little. Three reps, rest a little. Five reps, rest a little.	
Two reps, rest a little. Three reps, rest a little. Five reps, rest a little.	

Bird Dog: *Practice the movement on both sides, moving your knees closer together over time.*

Complex: *Do **two** repetitions of each exercise. Repeat for a total of three rounds.
Use a moderate weight.*

Row | Clean | Front Squat | Military Press | Back Squat | Good Morning

Round 1:		*Round 2:*		*Round 3:*	

High-Rep Back Squats *to Fifty*: *See page 104-105 for weight AND set/rep instructions.*

Record your weights and reps here: __________ | __________ | __________ | ________

Cool-down: *Record your personal cool-down plan of stretching or corrective exercises.*

____

____

Nutritional compliance (Y/N) _____ More protein _____ More fiber _____ More fish oil

WEEK SIX, SATURDAY — REST   DATE ______________________________

Shop, organize, prepare food

Nutritional compliance (Y/N) _____ More protein _____ More fiber _____ More fish oil

Other thoughts ____

____

____

WEEK SIX, SUNDAY — RECHARGE   DATE ______________________________

Your choice of 10-20 minutes of quality, low-intensity movement. Record your exercise choices and movement quality discoveries, and remember to note things to work on next *Recharge* day.

____

____

____

____

____

Nutritional compliance (Y/N) _____ More protein _____ More fiber _____ More fish oil

Other thoughts ____

____

Week Seven

Assess the program

Beginning weight, Monday ___________

Please review the assessment questions on page 54 before Monday, definitely before deciding where to take your training this week. Use the following pages to make good notes on your thoughts of the past six weeks. This may not seem important to you today, but next year when you decide to try this program again, you'll be very happy to have thorough notes on what worked and what did not.

If you honestly look over the six weeks, what parts worked? Did one tweak do better than all of the others for you? It might not be a bad idea to order them up from…

Best to Worst

________________ **Protein before bed**

________________ **Protein before the workout**

________________ **Creatine**

________________ **Protein upon arising in the morning**

________________ **Protein after the workout**

Also, take some time to think through the workouts. Yes, they're simple—

Four lifts (really only two)

One unchanging complex

High-rep squats

If you made progress, how complex does your future training need to be?

____

____

____

____

____

____

____

Notes:

Made in United States
Orlando, FL
11 November 2024